BREAST
BOTTLE
BOWL

THE BEST FED BABY BOOK

Anne Hillis & Penelope Stone

Illustrations by Kerry Millard

Angus&Robertson
An imprint of HarperCollins*Publishers*

This book is dedicated to
our children, Rachel,
Rowena and Sarah

and

Elizabeth and Felicity,
who showed us how
to put the theory
into practice!

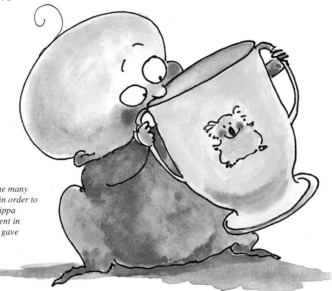

ACKNOWLEDGEMENTS

*We would like to thank Geoff Hillis for the many
hours spent deciphering our scribblings in order to
type our manuscript. Thanks also to Philippa
Sandall for her support and encouragement in
writing this book, and to all parents who gave
us the inspiration by asking a lot of
questions they couldn't find the
answers to.*

Angus&Robertson
An imprint of HarperCollins*Publishers,* Australia

First published in Australia in 1993 by Bay Books
This Angus&Robertson edition published in 1996
Reprinted in 1997
by HarperCollins*Publishers* Pty Limited
ACN 009 913 517
A member of the HarperCollins*Publishers (*Australia) Pty Limited Group

Text copyright © Anne Hillis and Penelope Stone 1993
Illustrations © Kerry Millard 1993

HarperCollins*Publishers*
25 Ryde Road, Pymble, Sydney, NSW 2073, Australia
31 View Road, Glenfield, Auckland 10, New Zealand

National Library of Australia Cataloguing-in-Publication data:

Hillis, Anne.
   Breast, bottle, bowl.
   ISBN 0 207 19004 6.
   1. Cookery. 2. Children–Nutrition. 3. Cookery (Baby foods).
   4. Infants–Nutrition. I. Stone, Penelope. II. Title.
641.5622

Editor: Kate Tully
Illustrator: Kerry Millard

9 8 7 6 5 4 3 2
99 98 97

Foreword

~

The foundations of good health are laid in the first years of life. It is in these years that you can help set your baby on the path to a life free of illnesses like heart disease, high blood pressure, certain cancers, stroke and diabetes. While these illnesses rarely strike before midlife, the processes that cause these 'lifestyle diseases' actually begin in childhood.

In the developed world, many children:
• are overweight or obese;
• have high blood cholesterol readings;
• are unfit and don't do enough regular exercise.

A high proportion of deaths in adults is related to what we eat and drink. While most of us are well aware of the links between nutrition and good health, most parents — especially first-time parents — are looking for special guidance.

For them, this book will be a welcome discovery. With its easy-to-read format and up-to-date information, it presents an overview of all the feeding issues that can crop up to confront parents. It gives clear answers to all those perplexing questions about what to serve and what not to serve. Best of all, it is loaded with simple and enjoyable ways to put this knowledge into practice, with its fuss-free, healthy recipes for children of all ages. *Breast, Bottle, Bowl* really takes the hard work out of feeding your baby and toddler. How I wish I had had a book like this when my first baby was born!

The authors, Anne Hillis and Penelope Stone, are experts in the field of feeding babies and children, being parents themselves as well as professional dietitians. Their clear advice has been gleaned from many years of working with babies, toddlers and children, and they have presented it in a way which all parents will find simple and easy to absorb.

Catherine Saxelby
B Sc, Grad Dip Nutrition & Dietetics, MDAA
Consultant Nutritionist

CONTENTS

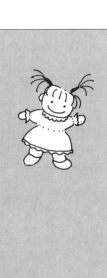

INTRODUCTION

~

As any parent knows — and may regret! — there are no schools where you can qualify as a parent before you become one. From the day a mother and baby arrive home from hospital, parents are involved in an intensive on-the-job learning experience, and this is true of feeding your child as much as of any other aspect of parenting.

We know exactly how you feel. We, too, are parents, but we have the advantage of also being qualified dietitians working in the baby health field. In this book we have combined our practical skills as mums with the dietary information you need so that you can keep this important part of parenting simple, enjoyable and stress-free.

We will show you how, by giving your child the 'right' food most of the time, the seemingly daunting task of ensuring a 'proper diet' will take care of itself.

You will find the book a handy guide both to what your child should be eating now and what he'll be up to next. It will take you all the way from your baby's earliest days to the increasingly adventurous palate of the pre-schooler and beyond.

When you've experimented with the ideas in our comprehensive recipe section, you'll be sure to have a good repertoire of meals to suit the age of your child; naturally the recipes can be prepared (sometimes with variations) for older members of the family, too. Of course, because we ourselves are mothers, all our recipes are quick and simple; we know we would rather be playing with our kids than spending all day in the kitchen!

Hygiene in the kitchen is vital to your family's well-being and is one aspect of feeding that needs to be taken especially seriously. Fortunately, good hygiene is easy when you know the ground rules. Please take time to read our advice on hygiene carefully.

Our A–Z Easy Reference covers many topics which, as parents, we are concerned about from time to time; keep this book in the kitchen and you will consult the A–Z many times over the coming years!

We know you will find *Breast, Bottle, Bowl* enjoyable as well as informative, and we hope it will help you give your child the best start in life — a healthy diet.

Anne Hillis
Penelope Stone

Postscript: We have used the term 'baby health nurse' to refer to those invaluable health professionals who go by different names all around the world, and we use 'he/him' when referring to babies and children, in order to avoid confusion with their mothers. We trust readers will agree that this is less cumbersome to read than repeated use of 'he/she' and 'him/her'. We have five daughters between us so you can be sure we are not biased in any way!

First things first

HEALTHY PARENTS HAVE HEALTHY CHILDREN

Starting to focus on the 'right' diet for our beloved offspring is a great way to re-examine our own diets too; it's unrealistic to expect our kids to develop good eating habits if we don't have them ourselves.

If parents eat well, keep only healthy food in the house and enjoy the energy and vitality which good eating brings, then they are doing themselves a favour as well as setting the best example they can to put their children on the path to a healthy life.

Like all things, eating well is easy when you know how. The table below shows the full picture of an adult's daily food needs. If it helps, photocopy this page and put it up somewhere in your kitchen, but you might prefer to just familiarise yourself with the overall requirements in each group. There's no need to become preoccupied with diet and make it into a chore. The important thing to remember is that if you include these foods in these quantities most of the time, you are well on the way to good health.

As you can see, on paper healthy eating is easy. However, in our daily lives it can become quite another matter.

DAILY NEEDS: ADULTS		
FOOD GROUP	**APPROXIMATE SERVING SIZE**	**MINIMUM NO. OF SERVES**
Bread and cereals Provide dietary fibre, protein, carbohydrates, vitamins, minerals, kilojoules	1 slice bread, ½ roll or muffin (include wholegrain or wholemeal varieties for dietary fibre) 2 cracker biscuits ½ cup (90 g/3 oz) cooked rice or pasta 1 bowl breakfast cereals (wholegrain and porridge are best)	4
Fruit and vegetables Provide dietary fibre, carbohydrates, vitamins (particularly Vit C), minerals, kilojoules	1 piece fruit ½ cup (125 ml/4 fl oz) fruit juice ½ cup (100 g/3½ oz) starchy vegetables (e.g. potatoes, peas, pumpkin, carrot, parsnip, sweet corn) 1 cup (120 g/4 oz) all other vegetables	4–6
Dairy foods Provide calcium, protein, vitamins, minerals, kilojoules Choose low fat varieties where suitable	¾ cup (200 ml/7 fl oz) milk 1 slice (40 g/1½ oz) cheese 1 tub (200 g/6½ oz) yoghurt	2 (3 for pregnant and breast feeding women)
Meat and substitutes Provide iron, protein, vitamins, minerals, kilojoules	1 small slice lean meat (veal, pork, beef, lamb, chicken, turkey) 1 medium fillet grilled or steamed fish 1 small can (100 g/3½ oz) salmon or tuna 1 egg 1–2 tablespoons peanut butter ¼ cup (40 g/1½ oz) nuts ½ cup (100 g/3½ oz) beans, lentils	2
Fats and oils Provide fatty acids, vitamins, kilojoules	1 tablespoon salad or cooking oil, salad dressing, mayonnaise, butter, cream, margarine or sour cream	1

Temptations, the weather, moods and other factors can all alter how we feel about our food.

One way to minimise the obstacles these present to your family's healthy eating is to develop a serious relationship with your shopping list. Always write out a list before you set foot in the supermarket and when you've made up the list, check to see that it contains food from each of the food groups in appropriate proportions. It's also a good idea to shop after a meal rather than when you're hungry, so that temptation doesn't overrule good intentions!

However well you may have been eating before, such a major event as the arrival of a baby is certain to have an impact on all aspects of a family's eating — on shopping and cooking as much as on mealtimes. When you're running yourself into the ground in the name of being a great parent, remember that a happy, healthy parent is much more likely to have a happy, healthy family.

Below are our tips for staying sane in this often unstable period, and ensuring that the main carer is cared for too.

---

10 hints for staying sane

1. Eat small, regular meals or nutritious snacks such as fruit, milk shakes, cheese and crackers or breakfast cereals with milk.

2. Accept all offers of help with household chores.

3. Take the phone off the hook when you are breast feeding or bottle feeding. This special time with your baby deserves your undivided attention.

4. Rest when your baby is sleeping.

5. If people ask what they can do to help, ask them to prepare a meal.

6. In the weeks before your baby is born, cook double quantities at each meal and freeze the extra for those early hectic weeks.

7. Write a list of daily and weekly chores and decide with your partner who will do what.

8. If anyone asks, a great gift is a nappy service for the first month (even longer if possible). It gives you more time for rest and the more enjoyable aspects of parenting!

9. Stock up on basic foods (rice, pasta, canned foods and so on) before your baby is born so that you only need to get a few items such as fresh meat and vegetables to make a meal.

10. Relax and enjoy your new baby and to hell with everything else! Your baby will only be tiny for such a short while.

CHAPTER ONE

IN THE BEGINNING

The all-milk diet

Breast feeding: The perfect meal every time

What comes beautifully packaged, is ready to serve and tastes terrific (to a baby, that is)? Of course it's breast milk. Nature's convenience food is designed to suit all babies.

WHAT'S SO GOOD ABOUT BREAST FEEDING?

For baby

1. Breast milk is the very best food your baby can get at this stage. It contains everything he needs until he's ready to expand his diet.
2. Breast milk is easily digested and absorbed. Remember that his little body is very immature.
3. Breast milk protects him from infection and it's also thought that it can protect him against the early development of allergies.
4. The composition of the milk changes to suit your baby.

For mum

1. It helps you get back into shape! The extra fat gained during your pregnancy is used up as energy during breast feeding.
2. Hormones released during feeding will help to contract your uterus back to its pre-pregnancy size and position.
3. There is the added bonus of no period when fully breast feeding — but this does not mean you are unable to fall pregnant!
4. Breast milk is ready to serve — no mixing, warming or waiting, and you don't have the extra work of sterilising bottles and teats.
5. It gives you time to enjoy your baby.

HOW IT WORKS

Breast milk first appears in the form of colostrum. Colostrum is very high in protein and minerals and particularly in antibodies, and it is very important that a newborn baby gets this precious fluid. Breast milk proper is produced by hormone changes in your body, usually two to five days after the birth.

Milk production is a continuous process, stimulated by the baby sucking at the breast. The composition of milk changes during the feed: the 'fore' milk at the beginning of a feed appears thin and watery while the later 'hind' milk is richer in fat. Some babies settle better after a feed if fed only from one breast because the feed is higher in hind milk and hence fat, so they feel more satisfied.

Milk is formed in glands at the back of the breasts. You can feel these as lumps when they are full of milk. Ducts lead from the glands into 15–20 sacs behind the nipple. When the baby suckles at the breast, a hormone is released which stimulates the milk to flow through the sacs to the nipple and into your baby's mouth: this is called the 'let-down reflex'.

GETTING STARTED

Start as soon as you feel up to it after the birth. The feel of your nipple on the baby's mouth will stimulate him to open it. He will get a small amount of colostrum from each breast and you will get the stimulation needed to produce milk.

One of the biggest problems in the early days of breast feeding is sore nipples, and one factor which can cause and aggravate this is poor position of your baby at the breast. You may feel comfortable sitting in a chair or in bed, or

lying down. Placing a pillow on your lap helps to raise your baby to the right level.

Place your baby on his side, with his chest against yours. Your baby will open his mouth when he feels the nipple on his lips. Allow him to take the nipple and most of the areola (the brown area around the nipple) into his mouth. As baby sucks you will feel the 'let-down reflex' as the milk begins to flow. If you are tense you can have difficulty experiencing this. Relax by having something to drink or eat, or a quiet read, and let nature take its course.

Rather than worrying about the duration of the feed, allow your baby to drink for as long as he wants. He will pause from time to time. If you need to remove him from your breast, put your finger into the corner of his mouth to break the suction. You can offer both breasts at each feed, but there are no rules for how long and how frequently your baby feeds.

Position, position, position!

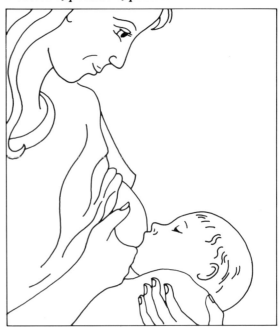

Position is essential for successful breast feeding. Good positioning ensures that the baby can suck productively, and helps to prevent sore nipples.

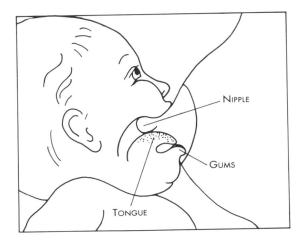

NIPPLE

GUMS

TONGUE

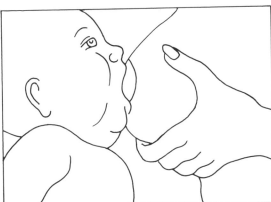

The baby's lips should pout to give a good seal over the areola. The baby's tongue is then able to roll and pump milk from the nipple. If the baby's lips roll in rather than out, he will tend to chew the nipple rather than suck, causing soreness.

Nutrients in breast milk

- Easily-digested protein for growth

- Fat in the right proportions, with essential fatty acids for growth

- Iron (in the same quantity as in cow's milk but absorbed five times better), important for healthy red blood cells and brain development

- Fluid — great for a thirsty baby

- Calcium for strong bones and teeth

- Protection from some stomach infections and some allergies

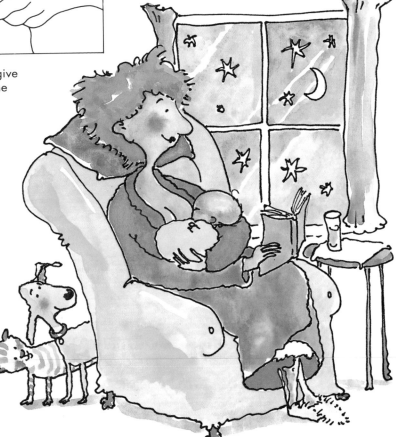

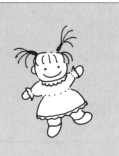

FOOD FOR BREAST FEEDING MUMS

Don't be surprised if you feel hungry all the time — breast feeding uses up a lot of energy. If you're starving, then just eat more, particularly fruits, vegetables, breads and cereals. Remember to also drink adequate amounts of fluid by drinking every time you feed your baby. You will probably feel more thirsty than usual.

Small frequent meals may suit you best. In each meal try to include reduced fat milk and dairy foods, fruit and vegetables and bread or cereals. Meat, chicken, fish, eggs, or meat substitutes should be included twice a day.

Copy the following meal plan and stick it on the fridge. During the day, check to see that you've eaten all you need.

Relief for engorged breasts: place cold cabbage leaves — yes, cabbage leaves — on them or place the leaves inside your bra, leaving a hole around the nipple.

BREAKFAST
Wholegrain/bran cereal
Reduced fat milk
2 slices toast with egg, baked beans or spreads
Tea/coffee

~

MORNING TEA
Glass reduced fat milk
1 piece fresh fruit

~

LUNCH
1–2 sandwiches with salad, lean meat and/or cheese
Reduced fat yoghurt and fruit
Tea/coffee

AFTERNOON TEA
Crackers/bread with cheese
Small glass fruit juice

~

DINNER
Small serve lean meat, chicken or fish
Potato, rice or pasta
3–4 varieties vegetables
Stewed fruit and custard

~

SUPPER
Hot milk drink

COMMON QUESTIONS ABOUT BREAST FEEDING

I have small breasts — will I be able to breast feed?

Size of breasts has little relevance in breast feeding. Each breast contains some 15–20 sacs which produce milk. These are stimulated by hormones in your blood to produce milk. Further stimulation will come from your baby sucking at your breast. Milk production is a continuous process.

How do I know if my baby is getting enough milk? Should I 'top him up' with formula just to be sure?

You will know if your baby is getting enough when he has at least six feeds per day (under 6 months) and is gaining weight satisfactorily. The number of wet nappies (about six per day) is also an indication that your baby is getting enough.

The baby's sucking at your breast stimulates further milk production, so just wait a few minutes and offer him the breast again. Extra feeding should provide enough stimulation to increase your milk production to meet your baby's increased growth needs.

In fact, topping up with formula is generally not recommended as it will decrease your breast milk supply because of the reduced stimulation. Topping up your baby with formula is actually the beginning of the weaning process from breast to bottle.

My milk is very thin and watery — is it still good enough for my baby?

Milk changes during a feed — at first it may be thin and watery but as the feed progresses it will appear richer. The composition of breast milk varies from woman to woman, during a feed and over the breast feeding period. If your baby is gaining weight well, your milk is just fine.

I find breast feeding difficult because of sore nipples. What should I do?

Sore nipples usually mean poor position of your baby at your breast. Check to see that your baby is taking in all the brown nipple area into his mouth. You may find 'air drying' your nipples after a feed will also help. If the condition persists, contact the Nursing Mothers' Association, La Lèche or similar organisations which help with breast feeding, or speak to your baby health nurse.

How often and for how long should I feed my baby? Sometimes it seems that I spend all day feeding him.

At first you may feed every 2–4 hours around the clock. While this is very tiring, the extra feeding will stimulate your supply and after a few days your baby will settle into a regular pattern. Remember, however, that what's 'regular' for other babies may not be regular for your baby — allow him to set his own pace.

When do I give up the 2 am feeds?

Most babies begin to give up the night feed at about six weeks, but some continue for longer. Try to go to bed immediately after the evening feed, to get maximum sleep before being woken again.

Won't breast feeding spoil my figure?

Nine months of pregnancy will have more effect on your figure than breast feeding; in fact breast feeding uses up the extra fat stored in pregnancy, so it actually helps your figure. Be realistic, though, about getting back into shape — if it took a few months to go out it will take a few months to come back in again!

I always seem tired — perhaps breast feeding is taking too much out of me and I should give up?

Be strict about getting some rest when baby rests, and look at your diet. Write down everything you eat during one day and compare it with the menu plan on the opposite page. Tiredness is unlikely to be due to breast feeding alone.

I'm going back to work, but I really would like to continue to breast feed. What should I do?

Express milk from each breast after each feed when at home, and store it in your refrigerator. Alternatively, feed the baby in the morning, after work and evening, and provide the carer with formula for the times you are not available.

Are there any foods I should avoid when I'm breast feeding?

Some mothers find that certain foods seem to upset their babies, such as spicy or 'windy' vegetables (cabbage, broccoli, Brussels sprouts, onion). Provided you still eat a good variety of foods, it is fine to cut out a few foods which seem to upset you or your baby. Of course, you should also avoid smoking and alcohol and use only drugs prescribed by your doctor.

Sometimes my baby goes for days without a dirty nappy. Does this mean he is constipated?

Some babies have a dirty nappy after every feed, others may go for a week without one. Both situations are normal.

How long before I give foods other than just breast milk?

Because your baby's digestive system is delicate, it is not designed to cope with foods other than milk much before four months. He will let you know when he's ready by not settling quickly after a feed and making chewing type movements with his mouth. If you offer him something on a spoon and he 'wolfs' it down, then you know it's time! (See Chapter Two: *Time to expand the menu.*)

Myths and messages about breast feeding

BABIES SHOULD BE FED EVERY FOUR HOURS

Babies should be fed when they are hungry. Sometimes this might be every two hours.

DAIRY FOODS CAUSE COLIC

The causes of colic are largely unknown. Dairy foods are important for calcium in a feeding mother's diet and should not be avoided.

TOO MUCH COFFEE DRIES UP YOUR MILK

Frequent sucking at the breast is what stimulates your supply. Caffeine can transfer in small quantities to breast milk but it is not a problem in moderation (about four cups of coffee per day).

YOU NEED TO DRINK LOTS OF FLUID TO BOOST YOUR SUPPLY

You will naturally be more thirsty, particularly once you are established in your breast feeding. If you produce 1000 ml (35 fl oz) of breast milk you will need extra fluids, but it is the suckling by the baby which will most effectively boost your supply.

AVOID ORANGES, CHOCOLATE AND GREEN VEGETABLES

While some foods seem to upset babies, it is important to include a variety of foods and to avoid a large amount of one particular food — avoid the chocolate binge!

Bottle feeding: Top class nutrition off the shelf

Some mothers decide to change from breast to bottle feeding soon after the birth, others after several months when the baby is still too young for a cup. The decision to give up breast feeding is often an emotional one already, and on top of that there are still people who will make a mother feel guilty, inadequate and downright worried about whether her baby is getting the right nutrients. This is both unfair and unnecessary.

Undoubtedly, breast milk is the very best food for a baby, but you can be assured that all infant formulas available in our stores are governed by very strict standards for their composition and safety and are therefore highly nutritious. Bottle feeding should not be regarded as a poor or second-rate alternative.

And contrary to what you might hear, the closeness and bonding experienced with breast feeding can also be experienced with bottle feeding. There's no reason you can't hold your baby close, provide plenty of eye contact and talk gently to him, just as you would when breast feeding.

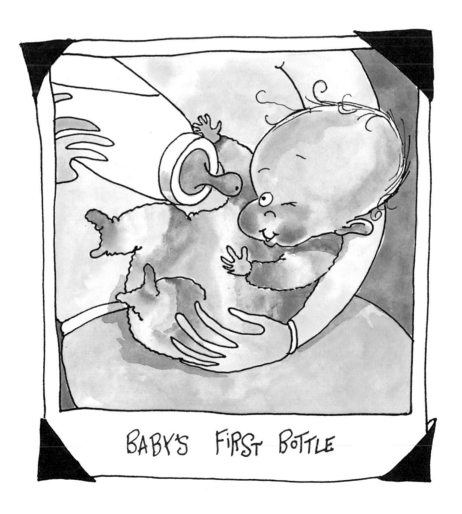

BABY'S FIRST BOTTLE

COMMON REASONS FOR CHANGING OVER TO BOTTLE FEEDING

1. Not enough milk.
2. Baby not gaining weight.
3. Baby feeding too often (every 1–2 hours). Some mothers find this so exhausting that the whole family becomes unhappy.
4. Breast problems such as inverted nipples, infection, engorgement or leaking breasts.
5. Returning to work, coupled with difficulty in expressing milk or no desire to express.
6. Fatigue coupled with poor self image — you can wear anything as long as it's accessible from the front!
7. Dislike of having baby always clinging to you — some of us need more personal space.
8. Partner unable to help with breast feeding but could help with bottle feeding.
9. Demands of other small children making it impossible to enjoy breast feeding.

INFANT FORMULA OR COW'S MILK?

An infant formula must be used instead of cow's milk as the main milk source for the baby's first 9 months and preferably 12 months. The reasons for this are:

• cow's milk is a poor source of iron and it's use may lead to iron deficiency anaemia;

• blood loss from the gut has been found in some children fed whole cow's milk before 12 months of age;

• cow's milk has too much protein (three times that of breast milk), sodium (three times that of breast milk), calcium and phosphorous — this puts a great strain on young kidneys to get rid of the extra protein and minerals as waste;

• cow's milk lacks vitamins A, C, and E; and

• cow's milk lacks essential fatty acids.

Cow's milk can be used in the preparation of solid foods (cereal, custards, sauces) from 4 months of age, provided it is boiled. Boiling helps to soften the protein and make it more easily digested. Cow's milk should always be boiled until the baby is at least 9 months old.

WHAT'S IN FORMULA?

Most infant formulas are based on cow's milk which has been modified to bring it closer to the composition of breast milk, the 'gold standard' for babies. Vitamins and minerals, vegetable oils and whey protein have been added, so there is no need to give your baby further vitamin and mineral supplements. All infant formulas must comply with the strictest nutritional and hygiene standards specific to each country.

Infant formula can be divided into two types:

1. those that are predominantly curd-based, as is cow's milk, and
2. those that are predominantly whey-based, as is breast milk.

Curds and whey are proteins of milk. Curds (or casein protein) are formed when milk mixes with acid, such as the acid in the stomach. Curds can be tough and hard to digest, particularly if the milk has not been treated.

Whey is the watery fluid left when the curds have been removed (remember junket?). It is easily digested, low in fat and protein and high in lactose (milk sugar), so it is quite sweet. Whey also contains a few minerals. The whey used in infant formulas is demineralised to give the formulas a mineral level similar to that of breast milk.

Breast milk contains approximately 60 per cent of its protein as whey and 40 per cent as curds, while cow's milk contains only 18 per cent as whey and 82 per cent as curds.

While both types of formula are suitable for a baby from birth, the whey-predominant ones are preferable as they are closer to breast milk.

All infant formulas must contain added iron. This is always at a higher level than in breast milk to allow for poorer absorption (breast milk iron is very efficiently absorbed).

Iron is one of the most important minerals in the baby's diet. It is required for getting the oxygen to body tissues where it is needed to produce energy. In muscles, iron helps produce energy for movement. Iron is also important for the brain. Recent research has linked iron deficiency to behavioural problems, learning difficulties and hyperactivity.

A baby is born with enough iron stores to last 4–5 months; after this it is very important that the baby's diet provides iron. Infant formulas now on the market contain different iron levels. Those with a lower level allow for the baby's in-built stores and are suitable only during these 4 months.

WHICH FORMULA?

Anyone would be forgiven for not knowing where to start when selecting an infant formula.

If you decide to bottle feed while still in hospital, you will be given advice on the most suitable formula, how to sterilise the bottles and how to prepare the formula correctly.

However, if you decide to bottle feed at a later stage you will need to consult your baby health nurse, doctor or dietitian for advice. That's because under the World Health Organisation (WHO) Code of Marketing Breast Milk Substitutes (see page 20), infant formula manufacturers are not allowed to advertise, promote or sample their formula directly to mothers, so you won't be able to pick up a magazine and compare advertisements for formulas. Formula manufacturers show their products to health professionals only, who will then pass on the necessary information. However, the following tables will also help you find your way through the many types of formula available.

FORMULAS SUITABLE FROM BIRTH		
FORMULA TYPE	CHARACTERISTICS	EXAMPLES*
Whey-predominant	Closest to breast milk Best for newborns Suitable from birth to 12 months (except†)	S-26 (GOLD CAP SMA) Wyeth NAN 1 Nestlé KARICARE INFANT FORMULA Douglas Pharmaceuticals ENFALAC ENFALAC REDUCED IRON† Mead Johnson (suitable to 4 months)
Curd-predominat	Suitable from birth, and for baby not satisfied on a whey-predominant formula Usually cost less than whey-predominant formulas	SMA (WHITE CAP SMA) Wyeth LACTOGEN Nestlé ENFAMIL Mead Johnson

* The name given first is the product name used in Australia. Where the same product is called by a different name in other countries, if available, that name is given in brackets.

FORMULA TYPE	CHARACTERISTICS	EXAMPLES*

Follow-on	Based on cow's milk
	Suitable for babies between
	    6 months and 2 years
	Have higher protein and mineral
	    content than formulas suitable from
	    birth, so *must not* be used for newborns
		S 26 PROGRESS (SMA PROGRESS)
		    Wyeth
		NAN 2 Nestlé
		ENFAPRO Mead Johnson
		KARICARE FOLLOW-ON
		    MILK Douglas Pharmaceuticals

* The name given first is the product name used in Australia. Where the same product is called by a different name in other countries, if available, that name is given in brackets.

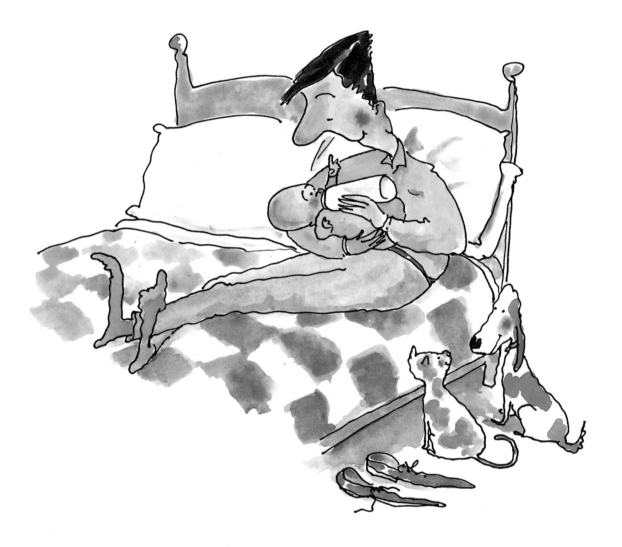

FORMULA TYPE	CHARACTERISTICS	COMMON REASONS FOR USE	EXAMPLES *

Soy	Made from soy beans
	Cow's milk-free
	Vitamins and minerals added
	Fat meets baby's needs
	Protein slightly higher
	  than breast milk
	Free of lactose (milk sugar)
	Carbohydrate is sucrose,
	  corn syrup solids or a mix
	  of both
	Suitable from birth
		Cow's milk protein intolerance
		Lactose intolerance
		After gastroenteritis
		Colic
		As a preventive against
		  allergy/skin reactions
			INFASOY (WYSOY)
			  Wyeth
			ISOMIL Abbott
			PROSOBEE and
			  PROSOBEE WITH
			  REDUCED IRON
			  Mead Johnson
			KARICARE
			  SOYA INFANT
			  FORMULA
			  Douglas
			  Pharmaceuticals

NOTES

The need for such formulas has been questioned by paediatric gastroenterologists for several reasons:
• There is a high intolerance to soy in babies who are also intolerant to cow's milk.
• After gastroenteritis when the gut is damaged, it may not be wise to introduce another foreign protein. Sucrose content may also be a problem.
• Sometimes iron and zinc may not be well absorbed.
• Soy formulas have high aluminium levels. While these have been lowered over the years, they are still higher than in breast milk and cow's milk-based formulas. The long-term effects of these higher levels are unknown. (See *Aluminium* in A to Z Easy Reference.)

Soy drinks are unsuitable for babies and must not be confused with soy formula. A soy formula must be used for babies up to 12 months; some health professionals recommend formula for up to two years. (See *Soy milk* in A to Z Easy Reference.)

Low lactose	Made from cow's milk in
	  which approximately
	  99 per cent of lactose has
	  been broken down to
	  glucose and galactose
	Similar to breast milk
	Suitable from birth
		Lactose intolerance
		  following gastroenteritis
		Chronic diarrhoea
		Colic-type pains
			DE LACT INFANT
			  Sharpe Laboratories
			OLAC Mead Johnson

NOTES

• Free of soy protein and lactose, so preferred following gastroenteritis and in lactase deficiency.
• Lactose is broken down more than by using enzyme (lactase) tablets or drops added to breast milk, or regular infant formula.

Goat's milk	Made from goat's milk with
	  composition similar to breast
	  milk
	Contains added vitamins
	  and minerals
	Carbohydrate is lactose
	Suitable from birth
		Cow's milk protein intolerance
		  in those who can tolerate it
		Alternative to cow's milk-
		  based formulas — said to be
		  more easily digested
			KARICARE
			  GOAT'S MILK
			  FORMULA
			  Douglas
			  Pharmaceuticals

NOTES

• Some babies can take goat's milk for cow's milk protein allergy, but most will not because goat's and cow's milk have similar proteins. Hence for most babies (about 65 per cent), goat's milk is not a suitable substitute.
• As it contains lactose, it is unsuitable for use in lactose intolerance and following gastroenteritis.
• Regular goat's milk (not formula) must not be used for babies less than 12 months. Compared with breast milk it lacks adequate amounts of folic acid and vitamins B12, C and D. Unpasteurised goat's milk should not be given to children.

* The name given first is the product name used in Australia. Where the same product is called by a different name in other countries, if available, that name is given in brackets.

The WHO Code of Marketing Breast Milk Substitutes

This Code was adopted at the 34th Session of the World Health Assembly in May 1981. It was a response to the decline in breast feeding in third world countries which resulted in many babies dying because mothers could not afford to buy enough formula or to prepare and store it correctly. While such problems do not generally apply to more developed countries, many governments have implemented the Code which specifies that breast feeding is promoted by all health professionals as the best way to feed a baby. The Code has ensured a high rate of breast feeding because women have access to adequate help, advice and support.

The Code does, however, recognise that those mothers who decide to bottle feed should be given good information and support.

THE CODE STATES THAT:

• infant formulas cannot be advertised or sampled directly to mothers;
• infant formulas should only be used on the advice of a health professional;
• labels must include a statement about the superiority of breast milk;
• labels must show the ingredients; and
• labels must provide instructions on the preparation and storage of the formula and carry warnings about the dangers of poor preparation.

PRACTICAL TIPS FOR BOTTLE FEEDING

There is no right or wrong time to start. Always discuss your decision with your hospital sister, baby health nurse, dietitian or doctor.

For some, changing from breast to bottle can be an easy transition while for others it is fraught with difficulties. Refusal of bottle and teat can be emotionally trying for any mother.

While some mothers find it best to gradually replace each breast feed with a bottle feed, others find it easier to go to the bottle 'cold turkey'. It should be noted, however, that this latter way can cause you difficulties with engorged breasts. If your baby refuses the bottle, you may need to try a different teat — it is usually not the formula which is disliked. Talk to your baby health nurse about any problems you encounter. (Depending on their age, some babies could be best going from the breast straight to a cup and by-passing the bottle. See page 25).

WHAT DO YOU NEED?

Bottles

If starting from birth you will need at least six. From 7 months, three to four will suffice. Choose 250 ml (8 fl oz) bottles for milk, but also purchase one or two smaller bottles. These are great for water and diluted juice.

Teats

You will need between four and six teats. Rubber and silicone teats are both suitable, although you will find that rubber ones will not last as long. Their lifespan is only about eight weeks, as they do not withstand heating well and your baby's acidic saliva will break them down.

Silicone teats are transparent, pliable, and can be repeatedly boiled and sterilised without deterioration. Silicone is an inert material and is safe, odourless and colourless. It is easy to see when a teat is blocked. Silicone teats are better value for money as they could last for the duration of bottle feeding unless a child chews them.

Vinyl teats are also available but not recommended. They cannot withstand temperature extremes through heat sterilising and easily lose shape.

Teats come in two basic shapes: conventional and orthodontic. Which one you use depends largely on trial and error. Selecting a teat for a baby who is being weaned from the breast can often be difficult and frustrating. If the baby is using a dummy, select a teat the same shape.

The conventional shape is usually cheaper than the orthodontic, very functional and performs well. The orthodontic shape replicates a mother's nipple when baby sucks. Some babies take in less air with this shape. The milk is spread over the baby's mouth rather than being squirted down the throat. The orthodontic teat is designed to enhance oral development.

The other consideration when selecting a teat is flow rate. Flow rate is determined by the size of the hole in the teat and you need to select the rate corresponding to the age of your baby. Holes too small for his age can cause wind, while holes too large can make the baby gag. As a general guide to flow rates:

Slow: 0–3 months
Medium: 3–6 months
Fast: 6–18 months

Change flow rates gradually.

Sterilising

All bottles and teats must be sterilised until the baby is a year old. This helps prevent illness.

1. Wash your hands and make sure your kitchen bench is clean.
2. Always make sure that bottles and teats are thoroughly clean before sterilising. You will need a bottle brush to clean effectively.
3. Bottles can be sterilised by boiling, steaming or by anti-bacterial solution or tablets. There are special sterilising systems on the market which are initially quite expensive but can be a worthwhile investment. If sterilising by boiling, follow the directions found on all infant formula labels. If using an antibacterial solution or tablets, follow the directions on the pack. Discard solution after 24 hours.
4. Do not rinse sterilised bottles before adding formula; a small amount of sterilising solution left in the bottle will not harm the baby.

Preparing formula

Always follow the manufacturer's directions exactly and use the scoop provided. Do not swap scoops from different formulas — they are different sizes and swapping can result in the baby getting too much powder or not enough. Always ensure the preparation area is clean, and that your hands are washed. Concentrate to ensure that you count scoops accurately.

While the labels will say bottles should be made up one at a time, it is also safe and more convenient to make up the day's supply of bottles in one go. Prepare directly into the bottle, as stated on the label. Do not use mixing bowls or spoons, as these may introduce unwanted bacteria. Keep formula for no longer than 24 hours.

Infant formula must be mixed with cool boiled water, not water straight from the tap. Water must be boiled for 5–10 minutes to make sure it is sterile. Bottled water is not sterile and is therefore not suitable for your young baby. Make sure you store made-up formula in the back of the refrigerator, as it is colder, not the door.

Warming formula

Most babies will prefer their milk warmed to body temperature. The recommended, best and safest method is to immerse the bottle in a container of hot water and let it stand for a few minutes, testing regularly on the wrist until the desired temperature is reached.

Many mums choose to microwave formula because it is quick and convenient and certainly the fastest way of getting a bottle ready for a crying baby. Care must be taken if microwaving. Timing is critical. Get to know your microwave and the time it takes to heat the bottle.

Formula will keep heating once removed from the microwave. Always shake the bottle thoroughly to mix the contents, because formula at the top of the bottle will be hotter than at the base. Always test formula on your wrist before giving it to your baby. Many a baby has been admitted to hospital with a scalded throat due to a hot feed. Remember when visiting friends that their microwave may be different from yours, so times will vary. Remember also that the microwaves in restaurants are often more powerful, so the time required will be much shorter.

There has been much publicity surrounding the safety of microwaving formula. A study showed that microwaving milk altered its amino acid pattern and the compounds resulting could possibly lead to kidney and liver damage as demonstrated in animals. However, the milk was heated in the microwave for 10 minutes which is far in excess of the time needed to heat formula — less than a minute.

If your baby does not finish all the formula in the bottle, throw it away (the formula that is, not the baby!).

COMMON QUESTIONS ABOUT BOTTLE FEEDING

Since I changed over to the bottle, my baby's dirty nappies have changed colour. Is this OK?

A breast fed baby has distinctive yellow 'poo', while that of a bottle fed baby is usually greeny black. This is due to the iron in the formula and is perfectly normal. Colour will also change as solids are introduced in the diet, probably to brown.

I think my baby is constipated. What should I do?

Constipation refers to poo which is hard and difficult to pass, not to frequency. Constipation is uncommon in breast fed babies. It is not unknown for breast fed babies to have only one dirty nappy in 10–14 days. In contrast, bottle fed babies usually have one every day. If you feel your bottle fed baby is constipated, try the following:

1. Check that you are making up the formula correctly. Are you using the right number of scoops to the right amount of water?
2. Check your baby's activity level. Active babies tend to be less constipated.
3. Try introducing prunes which contain a natural laxative (diphenylisatin). If baby is not yet on solids, try a teaspoon of undiluted prune juice. Older babies can have prune juice diluted in a bottle or a few puréed prunes on cereal or with custard.
4. Increase fluid intake. Give cool, boiled water. Try adding maltose to formula (Maltogen).

Always discuss your treatment with your baby health nurse. Suppositories and infant laxatives should only be used as a last resort and only under medical advice.

While high fibre diets including unprocessed bran are an effective treatment for the correction of constipation in adults, they are not recommended for babies less than 12 months old.

Do I still need to 'burp' my bottle fed baby?

Wind is air that babies swallow when they feed. All babies need to bring up this wind after a feed. Some will do this on their own if held or placed in the right position, others will need to be winded or 'burped'. If baby is very windy, check that the teat flow is right and that the cap containing the teat is not screwed down too tightly. Burp your baby during a feed, not just after it, to stop wind from building up.

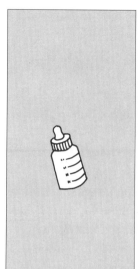

Remember bottles are for fluids only. Use for formula, water or diluted juices. Don't add food to bottles.

My baby seems to have diarrhoea. What should I do?

This can be a life-threatening situation for babies and it is most important you always see your doctor. See *Diarrhoea* in A–Z Easy Reference.

Should I put my baby to bed with the bottle?

While many parents will tell you your baby will sleep better if you put him to bed with a bottle — don't! The problem is that milk sits around the sleeping baby's teeth and bacteria in the mouth ferments the milk sugar into acid, causing tooth decay. First teeth are vulnerable to decay because new enamel is immature. At night, baby's saliva flow is reduced so that the natural self-cleaning action of the mouth is decreased, therefore decay is more likely. The same will occur if a baby is put to bed with a juice bottle, or even if he falls asleep during a breast feed. Encourage your baby to go to sleep with a cuddly toy, blanket or dummy for comfort instead.

My baby vomits after each feed. Is he sick?

This is a common problem and the amount of feed brought up varies from a lot to just a dribble. Vomiting can be caused by a weak valve between the oesophagus and the stomach and is called 'oesophageal reflux'. Babies usually grow out of this condition as the valve strengthens. If baby is vomiting to the extent that he is not gaining weight, it is important to consult your baby health nurse.

Some suggestions for dealing with a 'sicky' baby:
• Handle baby gently after a feed.
• Give small, frequent feeds using a slower teat.
• Feeds may need to be thickened (consult your baby health nurse).
• Raise the baby's mattress by putting a rolled pillow/blanket underneath it.
• Check that his formula is made up correctly.

My friends say their baby's formula is the best available — should I change over?

If your baby is happy and thriving on a formula suitable for his age group, it is best to leave him on it. Babies get used to their formula and can resist change. Changing formula unnecessarily can also lead to problems with preparation such as confusing scoops and scoop quantities. Always see your baby health nurse before changing formulas.

What do I need to know about colic?

See *Colic* in A–Z Easy Reference.

How can I make visiting easier when I'm bottle feeding?

The easiest way is to take cool boiled water in sterilised bottles and add formula powder when required. Sachets which contain the exact amount of powder for one feed are ideal for this. Warm the bottle in hot water in a cup (take boiled water in an insulated container if necessary). By taking the water and formula separately and mixing them only when needed, you reduce the risk of contamination.

An excellent alternative is the ready-to-feed bottles available from chemists and supermarkets. With these, you only need to warm the bottle and add a sterile teat. They are more expensive than formula made from powder, but very handy for occasional use.

If you do make up formula before visiting, it should be carried in a cooler box on ice. Sterile teats should be placed in a sterile container and kept cool.

When should I try a training cup?

By 6–8 months your baby should be able to swallow milk from a cup if it is held. By 12 months he can hold a cup and drink, so at about this time a training cup can be introduced. However, babies still prefer to have their milk from a bottle, deriving comfort and enjoyment from sucking. Use the bottle and training cup alternatively until baby is ready to forgo bottle for cup.

CHAPTER TWO

TIME TO EXPAND THE MENU

What to introduce when

Introducing your baby to the joys of dining

The decision to try foods other than breast milk or formula will largely be made by your baby. While you may think it's time and your baby health nurse will suggest it's time, your baby will make the final decision. He will let you know when he would like something extra.

Up until 4–6 months of age, all your baby's growth needs are met by breast milk or formula, but as he reaches that age he will start to indicate that he'd like something more. He has an energy gap which requires filling. You may notice that he doesn't settle as quickly after a feed, he starts to chew on his fists and toys and he even starts watching you eat with such intent that you feel guilty!

Don't fall into the trap of offering food earlier than this, in the hope that your baby will sleep longer through the night. Babies need frequent feeds when they are tiny, day and night, and there's nothing that will change that.

Apart from not needing the extra nutrition before 4 months, your baby also needs time to develop physically so that he can cope with solid food. You will have noticed that when your baby was very young he pushed his tongue forward: this is called the extrusion reflex and is important for sucking. Some mothers try to give solid food too early; when it is pushed out by the extrusion reflex, the mother decides the baby doesn't like that particular food and keeps trying others, with similar results. She then fears she has a fussy eater on her hands! In fact, the extrusion reflex does not disappear until 3–4 months, and only then can the baby take food from a spoon.

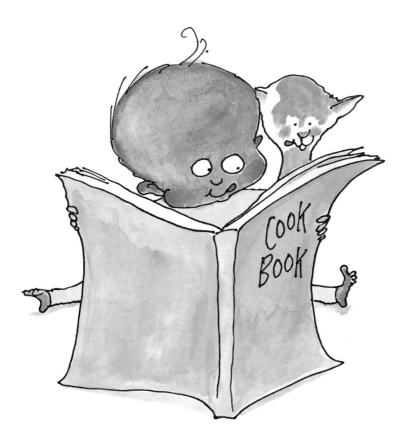

There is a lot of ongoing research into the best age to introduce solid foods. It seems that if they are introduced too early (before 4 months), not only is the baby unable to manage but there is a danger of allergy and perhaps obesity later on. On the other hand, your baby should be on solids by 6 months — by then breast milk or formula are inadequate for his energy needs.

SO, WHAT DO I DO?

It makes sense that a little baby needs a little bit of food on a little spoon.

1. Start with rice cereal. Mix a little with cool boiled water, formula or expressed milk until it is quite runny. If the mixture is too stiff, baby may not enjoy it — remember he is only used to liquids at this stage.

2. Try half a teaspoon after his milk feed and leave it at that, even if he eats it all.

3. Offer a little more each day until your baby gets used to it.

4. Once cereal is going well, try small amounts of puréed fruit and vegetables. Again, start with small quantities and gradually increase the amount to about two tablespoons. This might be over a few days or a few weeks, depending on how hungry he is. When introducing any new food, do it very gradually to check that there is no reaction.

5. Keep quantities small. How often we've heard of a baby trying a new food for the first time and just loving it, so he ate a cupful. After a few minutes he threw up the lot so the mother deduced that the baby had a reaction to the food. In fact he had just had too much at once. So take it slowly ... there is always tomorrow.

Rice cereal mixed with breast milk will become watery after a while because enzymes in breast milk 'break down' the cereal — it is still OK to use.

So how does it all work? The guts of the matter

Enzymes present in your baby's saliva begin the digestion of food. After swallowing, the food goes down the oesophagus into the stomach. A baby's stomach capacity is very small, so it makes sense that your baby needs to be fed often. The stomach is designed to store food, break it down into smaller particles and then send it on to the duodenum, the first part of the small intestine. At different stages of digestion various enzymes are produced in response to the type of food eaten. A special enzyme called rennin is present in a baby's stomach and is needed for milk digestion. Rennin 'sets' milk into a curd like sour milk, which is easily digested.

Most of the digestion of food occurs in the small intestine. Enzymes are produced to break down proteins, carbohydrates and fats. Nutrients are absorbed from the small intestine into the baby's bloodstream where they are used to produce energy.

Undigested food passes into the large intestine, where water and minerals are absorbed and the waste excreted.

When your baby is born, his intestine is sterile, but within a few hours of birth many bacteria may grow which are important for the digestion and absorption of milk. Breast fed babies have a different 'bacterial flora' from bottle fed babies. Once solids are introduced, the 'flora' changes.

Different foods affect your baby's 'poos'. Once the baby is on solids, you may notice flecks of undigested vegetables appearing. This is quite normal and as your baby grows and his digestive system matures, this will disappear.

Breast milk is served at the perfect temperature — body temperature — so use that as a guide to how hot a baby's food should be. Babies' mouths are easily burnt on food which is too hot. It is better to err on the side of caution and have it a little cold.

The best method of heating is to place the baby's food in a cup and stand it in a dish of very hot water. This way, the chill is off the food but there is no danger of it getting too hot. Microwaves are marvellous but as already advised with bottles, be certain to stir heated food very well and test the temperature on the back of your wrist (a very sensitive area).

Babies are born with four times more taste buds than we have as adults, so foods are very tasty to them and you shouldn't prepare your baby's food to suit your tastes. He hasn't acquired a taste for salt, so don't add it. Similarly, it doesn't make sense to add sugar — think of his future eating habits and his teeth. And don't add extra fat such as butter or margarine to foods. While your baby needs a certain amount of fat in his diet, he'll get all he needs from breast milk or formula and later on from cow's milk.

Once you have tried a range of different foods you will find that your baby is quite competent at taking food from a spoon. You can try rougher textures such as fork mashed vegetables and foods with soft lumps to encourage chewing. At first you might find that your baby gags: this is a natural reflex that prevents him from choking and once he has mastered (or spat out) the lumps he will manage very well. Don't worry if there are no teeth yet — babies chew very well with their gums.

Babies are not miniature adults

BABIES ...	ADULTS ...
... rely mostly on breast milk or formula for the first 12 months	... should rely mostly on bread and cereals, fruit and vegetables
... should have a diet fairly low in fibre for the first 12 months	... should include high fibre foods in their diets every day
... need whole milk products up to the age of 5 years	... need to change to reduced fat milk products

Once he has the small lumps under control, you can offer pieces of steamed vegetables, bread, meat and soft fruits as finger foods. Remember that food needs to be 'experienced' by your baby — worn, tasted, squished, dropped, rubbed in the hair and on mum or dad, thrown at the walls, used as a skin moisturiser and occasionally eaten. Good manners come later — this experimental time is an important part of your baby's development.

For more ideas on what to give your new little gourmet, see *First Foods* on page 60.

Introducing yourself to the joys of cooking for children

Well, it seems you've just had a baby and before you know it there's a new diner in the family. Doesn't time fly? Before your baby gets to the stage of eating a steak or a lasagne, you'll be a whizz at kids' cuisine. The following advice should come in handy.

First, always remember that cooking for babies and young children should not mean spending hours in the kitchen.

Please, keep it as simple as possible. Your child doesn't need elaborate meals and you don't need any extra stress. To make it easy on yourself, check that you have the following basic equipment soon after your little one starts on solids.
• A small steaming basket which fits all saucepan sizes. These are readily available at most supermarkets or hardware shops.
• A saucepan with a tight fitting lid
• Sieve and tablespoon, or special baby food sieve ('mouli')
• Fork for mashing
• Small plastic containers with tight fitting lids
• Child's bowls and small teaspoons
   Microwave ovens and food processors are just about standard equipment in most kitchens these days, but are certainly not essential.

Did you know ... a baby is born with about 12,000 taste buds? By the time we get to middle age, we have only 3000.

Your baby can gain 30 g (1 oz) a day for the first 3 months: that's some 2.7 kg (5 lb 10 oz), which may be more than he puts on in his whole second year.

Mummy, mummy! There's a germ in my soup!

We've all got germs (bacteria) in our kitchens, but we definitely don't need them in our food, especially with a young child in the house. Spoilage of food from bacteria is one of the greatest health hazards known to us, yet it is often ignored.

10 WAYS TO AVOID CLOSE ENCOUNTERS OF THE GERMY KIND

1. Wash your hands ... obvious isn't it? Always wash your hands before preparing food or feeding your baby and after changing his nappy.

2. Keep your kitchen utensils clean. Clean up as you go. This will not only save you time but help keep your kitchen free of germs.

3. Scrub your wooden chopping board under hot running water and then air dry.

4. Wear a clean apron when preparing food. Your family needs to be protected from your clothes, particularly if your baby is a dribbler or worse! Tie up long hair.

5. Buy the best quality foods, especially fruit and vegetables. Buy only enough for a few days at a time.

6. If in doubt, throw it out. Most leftovers can be stored in the fridge for up to 48 hours.

7. Always store prepared foods in covered containers at the back of the fridge. Never keep baby's formula in the door — this is the warmest part of the fridge, and it is difficult to keep below 4°C, and bacteria love temperatures between 4°C and 60°C.

8. Don't leave food sitting on the kitchen bench to cool. Place food in a shallow container, then place the container in cold water to cool it as quickly as possible before putting it in the fridge. Never put hot food into the fridge as it heats up all the other food, which will then go off more quickly.

9. Never defrost meat by placing it in the sink to thaw out during the day. Allow more time and defrost food in the fridge. Remember that if you feel comfortable at room temperature, so do bacteria. One bacterium can become 30 million within four hours at room temperature — a horrifying thought!

10. When reheating food from the fridge, bring to boiling point then cool down before serving. Even in the fridge, bacteria produce spores which also cause sickness, and most of these are destroyed by boiling.

WHAT ABOUT COMMERCIAL BABY FOODS?

Many mothers and health professionals are confused as to whether commercial baby foods are suitable for babies. Many arguments against their use seem to be offered by poorly-informed people.

Although we would never recommend a diet made up only of commercial baby foods, they certainly have their place in a diet of healthy, well-prepared meals. The huge variety offered in ready-to-serve units makes an excellent contribution to cooking for babies and children. They can be used alone as a meal or as part of a recipe.

Cost is often raised as an objection but, realistically, is it any less economical to open a jar than to prepare and cook half an apple?

Commercial baby foods are easily warmed by standing the can or jar in hot water for a few minutes, making sure that the lid has been pierced or loosened. If your baby requires only a small amount, spoon that amount into a cup and stand the cup in hot water; refrigerate the unused portion in a covered container immediately.

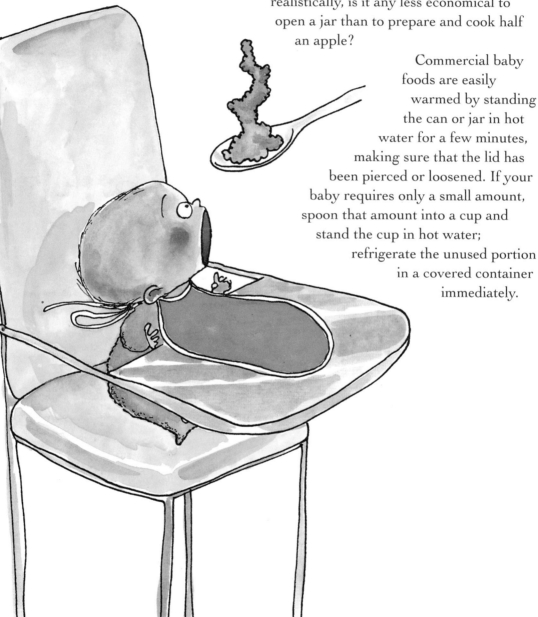

If you have fed your baby direct from a can or jar, throw away any leftover portion. The enzymes in your baby's saliva will make the food watery and germs from your baby's mouth will grow in the leftover food.

Specially formulated commercial infant cereal should always be used until your baby is around 12 months old. The manufacturers go to great lengths to ensure that the cereal is fortified with iron, is the right texture for each age group and is easily mixed. Infant cereal can be added to other foods such as fruit, vegetables, casseroles — it doesn't always have to be served at breakfast.

Commercial teething rusks are also very handy. You can make your own by drying out bread in the oven, but it is difficult to get the same degree of hardness. Rusks are for biting and chewing on, rather than a food in the true sense. Avoid teething rusks with added sugar.

Commercial baby foods are made from fresh fruits, vegetables, cereals and meat and are cooked according to very strict standards. Do you know the answers to these common questions?

COMMON QUESTIONS ABOUT COMMERICAL BABY FOOD

What about preservatives in commercial baby foods?

There are no preservatives in commercial baby foods. The canning process seals in the nutrients and the food is sterilised at very high temperatures. Provided no air can get in, these foods will store on your shelf for years.

How much salt is added to baby foods?

The natural sodium level is shown on the label. Some varieties do have added salt, so select those with none added.

Is sugar added to baby food?

Choose varieties with no added sugar. A small amount (about 4 per cent) in custards is acceptable

Is commercial baby food as nutritious as a home-cooked meal?

It is as nutritious as a well-prepared meal cooked at home without added salt, sugar or fat (butter, margarine, oil or cream).

FREEZING

It's as easy to cook enough for two meals as for one, so get into the habit of cooking enough to freeze some. It will save you hours! For example, when preparing puréed vegetables or fruit, cook an extra quantity and divide it into an ice cube tray, cover with plastic wrap and freeze. Once frozen, place the cubes in a freezer bag and store in the freezer. To heat these portions, place in the microwave or stand in hot water. You will notice that fruits and vegetables are a bit 'watery' after being frozen. This is quite acceptable — freezing causes it but the food is still safe and nutritious.

Commercial baby foods can also be frozen; again the texture is altered but the food is still safe to use.

What next? Life beyond purée

There is always confusion among parents about what foods to introduce when. To make it easy, we have prepared the tables on the following pages showing the approximate ages at which many different foods can be offered. There's also some useful information on the different food groups and on preparation.

Remember that texture is as important as the type of food — too much sloppy food once your baby can handle more lumps makes your baby lazy and doesn't encourage chewing, which is important for healthy tooth and jaw development and for speech later on.

BREAD AND CEREALS

This is a general term which includes all food and food products made from grains such as bread, rolls, pita bread, savoury biscuits, rice, pasta and breakfast cereals.

When cereal is introduced at 4–6 months, rice cereal is generally given as it is free of gluten (see *Gluten* in A–Z Easy Reference) and unlikely to cause any upsets for a baby. Other types of cereal are introduced later (see table). Infant cereals must, by law, be fortified with iron. They are also low in fibre compared with adult cereals. A baby's delicate gut does not require harsh cereal fibre. Fibre is very bulky and can 'fill up' your baby so that he doesn't have room for all the other food he requires. Fibre also interferes with the absorption of some important nutrients.

Preparation

Cereals are traditionally served with milk — breast milk, formula or boiled cow's milk for younger babies. Cereal can also be mixed with fruit purée or diluted fruit juice or cool, boiled water.

WHAT FOODS WHEN?: BREAD AND CEREALS			
AGE TO INTRODUCE	TYPE	SELECTION	PREPARATION
4–6 months	Rice-based infant cereal	Commercial varieties	Follow manufacturer's instructions
6–7 months	Wheat-based infant cereal	Commercial varieties	Follow manufacturer's instructions
	Bread	White varieties	Toasted, rusks
	Rice	White varieties	Boil/microwave as per manufacturer's instructions
	Pasta	White varieties	
8 months	Infant muesli	Commercial varieties	Follow manufacturer's instructions
	Bread	Wholemeal varieties (no grains)	Toasted, plain
10 months	Grains	All varieties	
	Adult cereal	Varieties without added salt and sugar	Add milk until mushy, or serve dry as a biscuit substitute
	Bread	Wholemeal, wholegrain	Toasted, plain
12 months	Breads, grains and cereals	All varieties	

FRUIT AND VEGETABLES

When offering a vegetable for the first time, serve a little on its own. Some babies like their vegies mashed together, others are more selective.

Babies love fruit and most fruits are well received after 8 months, although strawberry and citrus fruits can cause rashes in some children. When offering a fruit for the first time, give only a small quantity and wait a few days. There is always a temptation — especially if your baby loves a food — to give too much at first without knowing the consequences.

Use the following tables as guides only. Some babies can manage foods earlier, others later.

Preparation

Steaming and microwaving are the best ways of cooking vegetables and fruit. Prepare as close to serving time as possible as the vitamin content of these foods is considerably reduced when peeled, soaked or diced.

When steaming, place the steaming basket in a small saucepan containing half a cup of boiling water, add the vegetables or fruits which have been peeled, sliced and washed, replace the lid and steam until tender.

When microwaving, place vegetables or fruits in a microwavable container. Cooking and standing time should be according to the quantity of the food: check the times suggested for your particular oven.

Fork mash the cooked vegetables/ fruits or push through a sieve with a spoon. You may need to add a little boiled water or formula to thin down to the right consistency.

Do not add salt, sugar, butter or margarine. Your child doesn't need them and adding these can start a lifetime of bad habits.

After 6 months when your baby begins to feed himself, cut vegetables into chips or pieces, steam and offer as finger foods, because fingers are so delicious! Fruits will probably be best managed raw.

WHAT FOODS WHEN?: FRUIT			
AGE TO INTRODUCE	TYPE	SELECTION	PREPARATION
From 4 months	Apple	All varieties, crisp skin	Peel, dice, steam 20 minutes or microwave, mash.
		Commercial varieties	Open can or jar, serve cold or warm.
	Apricot	Ripe, firm, soft	Wash, remove stone, steam or microwave, purée.
		Commercial varieties	Open can or jar, serve cold or warm.
	Banana	Ripe, firm to soft	Peel, fork mash.
	Mango	Firm to soft, pink blush	Peel, fork mash.
	Peach	Ripe, soft yellow or white varieties	Peel, steam or microwave, mash.
		Commercial varieties	Open can or jar, serve cold or warm.
	Pear	Soft yellow or brown	Peel, remove core, slice, steam or microwave, fork mash.
		Commercial varieties	Open can or jar, serve cold or warm.

AGE TO INTRODUCE	TYPE	SELECTION	PREPARATION

From 8 months	Berry fruits
	  blackberry
	  blueberry
	  raspberry
	  strawberry
		Fresh or frozen	Fresh: wash, serve as finger foods.
			Frozen: defrost and serve.

	Cherry	Fresh, dark red, soft	Wash, remove pips, serve as finger food.
	Dried fruit	Currants, raisins, sultanas	Offer *small* amounts (6 to 8). Soak in water for ½ hour to soften, serve mixed with other fruit.
	Fig	Fresh (green firm skin, pink flesh) or dried	Fresh: give small amounts, mash. Dried: soak ½ hour in water, serve chopped with other fruits.
	Grape	Green, sweet varieties	Wash remove pips, serve a few at a time as finger food.
	Grapefruit	Yellow or pinkish skin	Peel, remove pith, cut into pieces, serve as finger food.
	Kiwifruit	Firm brown furry skin, green flesh with black pips	Peel, slice, serve as finger food.
	Mandarin	Firm, orange skin	Peel, remove pips, pith and 'strings', offer segments as finger foods.
	Melon honeydew	Firm, pale green skin, moist green flesh	Peel, slice, dice, serve as finger food.
	rockmelon (canteloupe)	Rough beige skin, firm to soft, orange to pink moist flesh	Peel, slice, dice, serve as finger food.
	Orange	Firm orange skin	Peel, remove pips and pith, offer segments as finger food.
	Nectarine	Firm yellow skin with red blush, yellow-green flesh	Peel, remove stone, slice, serve as finger food.
	Pineapple	Fresh: if spike pulls out easily, fruit is ripe Canned: with no added sugar varieties	Peel, dice, serve as finger food. Ready to serve diced or crushed.
	Plum	Dark red or yellow	Wash, remove stone. Stew gently 20 minutes, serve. Serve fresh as finger food (can be rather tart).
	Prune	Purple/black, moist, plump (these are dried plums.)	Remove stone, soak, serve as finger food — only one!
	Rhubarb	Red firm stalks	Wash, chop into lengths, stew, serve with stewed apple (a small amount of sugar is warranted here).

AGE TO INTRODUCE	TYPE	SELECTION	PREPARATION
4–6 months	Avocado	Flesh must feel soft under the skin when gently pressed	Peel, stone, fork mash, serve raw.
	Marrow	Firm moist flesh, no soft spots	Peel, cut into chunks, steam 15 minutes or microwave, fork mash.
	✓Potato	Firm red or white skin, no green skin	Peel, cut into chunks, steam 20 minutes or microwave, fork mash. Thin with boiled water or formula.
	✓Pumpkin	Yellow or dark green skin and firm yellow flesh	Peel, dice, steam 20 minutes or microwave, fork mash.
	Squash	Yellow skin and firm white flesh	Peel, dice, steam 15 minutes or microwave, fork mash.
	Swede	Purple and white skin firm white flesh	Peel, dice, steam 20 minutes or and microwave, fork mash.
	Sweet potato (kumera)	Firm yellow flesh	Peel, dice, steam 20 minutes or microwave, fork mash.
	Zucchini (courgette)	Dark green, firm to touch, white flesh with seeds	Wash, peel, cut into slices, steam 15 minutes or microwave, sieve.
6–7 months	Aubergine (eggplant)	Purple, firm, shiny surface, small, young fruit	Wash, cut in half. Place on lightly greased tray, bake in oven 40 minutes. Scoop out flesh, sieve.
	Beetroot	Choose small young beets	Wash, 'top 'n' tail'. Boil 30–40 minutes, sieve/purée.
	Broad bean	Firm green pods	Pod, steam 15 minutes, sieve/purée.
	Broccoli	Firm green heads	Wash, cut into flowerettes, steam 15 minutes or microwave, serve as finger food.
	Carrot	Crisp, young	Scrub or peel, wash, slice, steam 15 minutes or microwave, serve puréed or as finger food. *Note: never serve raw carrot to children under 3 years, unless grated.*
	Cauliflower	Firm white heads	Cut into flowerettes, wash, steam 15 minutes or microwave, serve as finger food.
	Celery	Crisp green sticks	Wash, cut into small strips, remove strings, steam 3–4 minutes or microwave, serve as finger food.
	Green bean	Young, crisp, green	Wash, cook whole if small or cut into strips, steam 5 minutes or microwave, serve as finger food. Steam 10 minutes to purée.
	Parsnip	Firm, white	Peel, wash, dice, steam 15 minutes or microwave, purée or fork mash.
	Pea	Fresh or frozen	Steam 10 minutes or microwave, mash.
	Spinach	Fresh (crisp leaves, dark green) or frozen	Fresh: wash thoroughly, chop, steam 5 minutes or microwave, purée. Frozen: steam 5 minutes or microwave.

AGE TO INTRODUCE	TYPE	SELECTION	PREPARATION
6–7 months	Silverbeet	Crisp leaves, dark green	Wash thoroughly, chop, steam 5 minutes or microwave, purée.
	Tomato	Fresh or canned Canned: purée or mash.	Fresh: finely dice as finger food.
	Turnip	Firm white flesh	Peel, dice, steam 10 minutes or microwave, purée or fork mash.
8 months	Brussels sprout	Small firm sprouts	Wash, cross cut stem, remove older outer leaves, steam 10 minutes or microwave, mash, chop or serve whole.
	Cabbage	Crisp leaves	Shred finely, wash, steam 6 minutes or microwave, serve as finger food.
	Leek	Smaller white with firm green leaves	Remove stem, cut into pieces, slice lengthways, separate sections under running cold water to remove any soil, slice, steam or microwave, chop.
	Lettuce	Fresh, crisp green leaves	Wash leaves thoroughly, pat dry on paper towel, shred very finely
	Onion	White	Remove skins, dice, steam 5 minutes or microwave, and serve or use as part of a dish. Note: small amounts of onion can be used earlier as part of other dishes.
	Sweetcorn	Fresh (small pale kernels) or canned (creamed)	Fresh: remove husks, place in boiling water for 3–5 minutes (overcooking makes corn tough and tasteless). Fresh uncooked corn requires a good set of teeth! Wait until 3 years. Canned: heat and serve or use as part of a dish.

WHAT FOODS WHEN?: MEAT

AGE TO INTRODUCE	TYPE	SELECTION	PREPARATION
6 months	Beef Lamb Pork Chicken Turkey	Lean, fresh	Casserole or roast, then purée or finely mince, mix with gravy or boiled water.
	Fish	Boneless fillets	Steam for 20 minutes or microwave, then mash, checking carefully for bones. Moisten with formula or boiled milk and add vegetables for the right consistency.

WHAT FOODS WHEN?: MEAT SUBSTITUTES

AGE TO INTRODUCE	TYPE	SELECTION	PREPARATION
6 months	Eggs	Yolk only	Well cooked
	Chick peas	Dried Canned	Soak overnight, boil until tender, mash. Mash
	Lentils	Dried	Soak overnight, boil until tender, mash.
8 months	Nuts	Peanut butter	*Never* give whole nuts under 5 years — always use as a paste.
	Seeds	Sesame Poppy Pumpkin	Tahini paste Sprinkle on foods. Grind, serve as a paste.
10 months	Eggs	Whole	Cooked whole egg, if tolerated.

WHAT FOODS WHEN?: DAIRY FOODS

AGE TO INTRODUCE	TYPE	SELECTION	PREPARATION
From 4 months	Yoghurt	Whole milk varieties	—
	Cow's milk	Whole	Boiled, small amount on cereal or in custard, sauces
	Custard	Homemade	Use boiled cow's milk and egg yolk only or custard powder.
		Commercial	Heat and serve.
From 6 months	Cheese	Whole milk varieties	Grated*
10 months	Cow's milk	Whole	Offer in a cup.

* Cheese is best offered grated at first as large pieces can stick to the roof of a baby's mouth and cause him to choke.

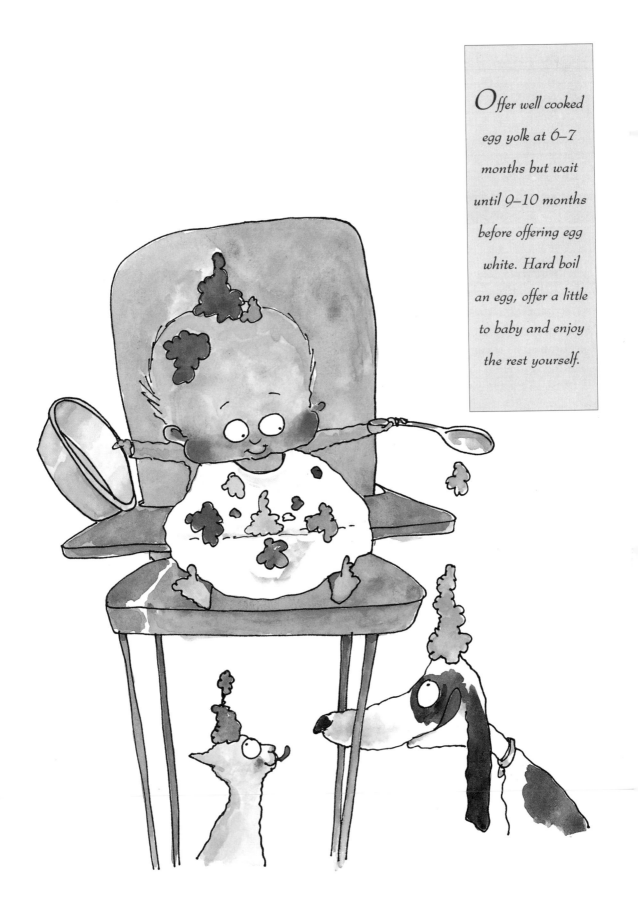

Offer well cooked egg yolk at 6–7 months but wait until 9–10 months before offering egg white. Hard boil an egg, offer a little to baby and enjoy the rest yourself.

Young vegetarians

People choose to follow a vegetarian diet for many reasons. Being vegetarian doesn't just mean avoiding meat; there are several different styles of vegetarian eating.

A *lacto-vegetarian* diet includes dairy foods as well as fruits, vegetables, breads, cereals, nuts and legumes but excludes meat, poultry, fish and eggs. A *lacto-ovo-vegetarian* diet also includes eggs.

A *fruitarian* diet consists of fruits and nuts only and is not suitable for children.

A *macrobiotic* diet involves various levels of food restriction and is not suitable for children as it cannot provide the essential nutrients they require.

A *vegan* diet avoids all foods of animal origin, including milk, cheese and eggs. It is difficult for a young child to eat the quantities of fruits, vegetables, breads, cereals, nuts and legumes otherwise required to provide energy for normal growth and development, so a vegan diet is not recommended for babies and young children. Nutrients at risk include fat, calcium, zinc and riboflavin.

Until 6 months, all babies are 'vegetarian'. After that, lacto-vegetarian and lacto-ovo-vegetarian diets can provide all essential nutrients.

Follow the guidelines for introducing solids as already discussed. After 6 months offer small quantities (1–2 teaspoons) of puréed lentils, legumes or smooth peanut butter. Remember that breast milk or formula is the main source of nutrients for your baby for the first 12 months.

Points to remember when feeding vegetarian children:

Energy

It is important to make sure your baby or young child has enough milk, whether it be breast milk, formula, cow's milk or soy milk. This should be the basis of his diet to provide adequate amounts of fat for energy. Fruits, vegetables, bread, cereals, nuts and legumes are bulky and can reduce the amount of food your child can eat. Offer milk, cheese and egg first in the meal, before your child becomes too full.

Protein

Animal proteins (meat, fish, chicken, eggs, milk, cheese) are important for growth. Plant proteins only help growth if mixed with certain other proteins to resemble the 'complete' protein found in animals. Some examples are: legumes mixed with bread or cereals (such as baked beans on toast); dairy foods or eggs mixed with bread, cereal, legumes or nuts (such as cereal and milk); bread or cereal mixed with nuts (such as peanut butter sandwich).

Iron

The best source of iron in the diet is meat. However, in a vegetarian diet other foods can provide iron:
- breast milk or formula for the first year
- iron-fortified infant cereal (you can continue to use these up to the age of 2 years)
- iron-fortified adult cereal after 10–12 months
- wholegrain breads
- legumes, lentils
- green leafy vegetables
- iron-fortified soy formula

It is important to include some fruit and vegetables containing vitamin C at the same meal, as the vitamin C improves iron absorption from plant foods.

Calcium

Breast milk, dairy foods, cow's milk or fortified soy milk in adequate quantities will ensure that your child has sufficient calcium.

Zinc

Animal foods are the best sources of zinc but a child on a vegetarian diet will receive adequate amounts from breast milk, cow's milk, fortified soy milk, eggs, dried peas and beans, wholegrain/wholemeal bread and cereals and nuts.

Vitamin B12

This is only found in animal foods (except for small quantities in fermented vegetable foods such as soy sauce). Dairy foods and eggs in your child's diet will provide adequate amounts of vitamin B12.

VEGETARIAN MENU FOR CHILDREN 1–5 YEARS

BREAKFAST	AFTERNOON TEA
Iron–fortified infant muesli	1 slice cheese
Milk or fortified soy drink	125 ml (4 fl oz) milk or fortified soy drink
1 slice wholegrain toast	
Peanut butter	
Small glass fruit juice	~
	DINNER
~	Cooked beans
	Vegetables
MORNING TEA	Stewed apples and yoghurt
125 ml (4 fl oz) milk or fortified soy drink	
Banana	~
	SUPPER
~	125 ml (4 fl oz) milk or fortified soy drink
LUNCH	
Egg sandwich	
Fruit salad	
Milk or fortified soy drink	

Our recipe section includes many vegetarian recipes suitable for all ages.

Fill a container with pieces of chopped fruit, sultanas and cheese and keep in the fridge. When your child needs a nourishing snack, he'll enjoy being able to help himself from his own 'snack pack'.

CHAPTER THREE

IS THIS NORMAL?

The link between development and diet

Ages and stages

The important information on the following pages shows the whole story of your child's development from birth to 5 years and how it relates to his food needs and eating habits. Use this information to see what you can expect now and what to prepare for next; it's the nature of bringing up children that just when you think you've mastered the stage they're at, they're moving on to the next one!

Note that the average heights and weights given here are derived from growth charts used for Australian children. The heights and weights of children are influenced by their parents' height and weight and also by ethnic background. Children from different ethnic backgrounds may have different average heights and weights to those of Australian children. Check with your baby health nurse.

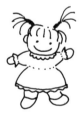

Ages and Stages: 0 to 4 months

AVERAGE WEIGHT

Boys
Birth: 3.2 kg (7 lb)
4 months: 6.6 kg (14 lb 9 oz)

Girls
Birth: 3.2 kg (7 lb)
4 months: 6.0 kg (13 lb 4 oz)

Average weight gain 150–200 g
(5–7 oz) per week

Growth spurts at 6 weeks and 3 months
Weight doubles by 4–5 months

AVERAGE LENGTH

Boys
Birth: 50.5 cm (20 in)
4 months: 63.7 cm (25 in)

Girls
Birth: 48 cm (19 in)
4 months: 62 cm (24 in)

DEVELOPMENT

- Hears normally
- Sees at close range
- Responds to mother's voice and smell
- Smiles at 4–6 weeks
- Sleeps well most of time
- Digestive system too immature to cope with foods other than breast milk or infant formula
- Small stomach capacity and immature kidneys
- Enzyme for milk digestion (lactase) is present
- Sucks well — tongue moves up and down
- Tongue pushes out food fed from a spoon (extrusion reflex)

DIET

- Only breast milk or infant formula are necessary for energy and nutrition
- Approximately 600 ml (21 fl oz) daily required at birth, 1000 ml (35 fl oz) daily at 4 months
- Takes 5–6 feeds per day every 3–5 hours
- Extra feeds may be required during growth spurts
- Solids not required at this stage — digestive system is too immature to cope. Early introduction may lead to allergy and obesity
- Cool boiled water can be given in addition to breast milk or formula in very hot, humid weather

TEXTURE AND FEEDING NOTES

Liquid milk diet only

SAMPLE MENU
At 4 months

5–6 feeds per day every
3–5 hours
(e.g. 6 am, 10 am, 2 pm, 6 pm,
10 pm and possibly 2 am)

Ages and Stages: 4 to 6 months

AVERAGE WEIGHT

Boys
4 months: 6.6 kg (14 lb 9 oz)
6 months: 7.8 kg (17 lb 3 oz)

Girls
4 months: 6.0 kg (13 lb 4 oz)
6 months: 7.2 kg (15 lb 14 oz)
Weight gain 150–200 g (5–7 oz) per week

AVERAGE LENGTH

Boys
4 months: 63.7 cm (25 in)
6 months: 68 cm (27 in)

Girls
4 months: 62 cm (24 in)
6 months: 66 cm (26 in)

DEVELOPMENT

- Holds head up — good control by 6 months
- Teething may have started
- Tries to talk
- Can hold rattle
- Extrusion reflex disappears — tongue moves back and forth to take food from spoon for swallowing
- Chewing movements appear at about 6 months even if no teeth are present
- Digestive system more mature
- Excited when sees food
- Milk becomes inadequate for energy requirements between 4 and 6 months, so it's time to introduce solids
- Iron stores built up during pregnancy are depleted by about 4 months

DIET

- Breast milk or formula is continued (not cow's milk):
4 months: 5 feeds (1000 ml/35 fl oz) daily
6 months: 4 feeds (900 ml/32 fl oz) daily
- Solid food introduced. Rice cereal is first (source of iron, easily digested, bland, unlikely to cause allergy)
- Single ingredient vegetables (potato, carrot, pumpkin, zucchini) introduced after 1–2 weeks, then single ingredient fruits (banana, apple, pear) and gels
- Small quantities of yoghurt, custard can be added
- Boiled cow's milk can be used in small quantities on cereal and to prepare solids, but not as main milk drink
- Juices diluted 50 per cent with water can be used if needed
- No sugar, salt, margarine, butter or oil added

TEXTURE AND FEEDING NOTES

- Strained or finely sieved at first, then roughly fork mashed
- Served cool or warm (always check temperature first, especially when microwaving)
- Small spoons and bowl used
- Hygiene vital during preparation
- For recipe ideas see *First Foods* on page 60
- Solids start at one meal daily then increase to 2–3 meals by 6 months, given after milk feed
- Honey, spinach and vegetable water avoided (see *Honey* and *Nitrates* in A to Z Easy Reference)

Breakfast
Breast milk or formula

AM
Breast milk or formula
1–2 tablespoons rice cereal

Lunch
Breast milk or formula
1 tablespoon mashed or puréed fresh fruit or ⅓ jar (40 g/1½ oz) strained fruit

Dinner
Breast milk or formula

1 tablespoon boiled/steamed vegetables mashed OR ⅓–½ (40–55 g/1½–2 oz) jar strained mixed vegetables

Before bed
Breast milk or formula (if needed)

Ages and Stages: 6 to 9 months

AVERAGE WEIGHT
Boys
6 months: 7.8 kg (17 lb 3 oz)
9 months: 9.2 kg (20 lb 4 oz)

Girls
6 months: 7.2 kg (15 lb 4 oz)
9 months: 8.6 kg (18 lb 15 oz)
Weight gains slow down to about 100 g (3½ oz) per week

AVERAGE LENGTH
Boys
6 months: 68 cm (27 in)
9 months: 72.5 cm (28 in)

Girls
6 months: 66 cm (26 in)
9 months: 70 cm (27½ in)

DEVELOPMENT
• Responds to name
• Sits without help
• Holds bottle
• Feeds himself finger food
• Holds small object with thumb and index finger
• Teething
• Chews lumpier food

DIET
• Three feeds of breast milk or infant formula (600–700 ml/21–24 fl oz) daily plus three meals
• Solid food can now be taken before milk
• Wheat foods can be introduced, e.g. infant mixed cereal can replace rice at 6 months, then infant muesli at 8 months
• Egg yolk can be taken from 6 months, egg white from 9 months
• Time to try:
minced beef, chicken, fish, pasta, rice, beans and lentils, grated cheese, teething rusks, toast/bread, finger foods
• Boiled cow's milk can be used on cereals, in yoghurts, custards, other desserts, sauces, but not as a main milk drink

TEXTURE AND FEEDING NOTES
• Roughly fork mashed, small lumps, commercial 'Junior' texture
• Salt, sugar and honey avoided, small amount of margarine and butter on bread
• Sausages, peanuts, raw carrots, hard nuts, whole peas and other foods that could cause choking also avoided
• Adult cereals too low in iron and too high in fibre and salt
• For recipe ideas see *More Tastes and Textures* on page 61

SAMPLE MENU At 9 months

Breakfast
2 tablespoons infant muesli
1 slice toast
Breast milk or formula

AM
125 ml (4 fl oz) diluted juice

Lunch
Stewed fruit and yoghurt
Breast milk or formula

PM
Diluted juice
1 rusk

Dinner
2 teaspoons lean meat, chicken or fish
½ cup (75 g/2½ oz) steamed
vegetables, diced or mashed

Before bed
Breast milk or formula (if needed)

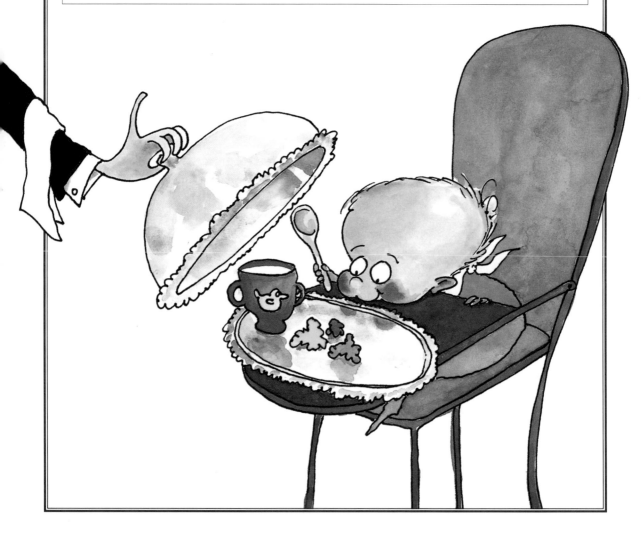

Ages and Stages: 9 to 12 months

AVERAGE WEIGHT
Boys
9 months: 9.2 kg (20 lb 4 oz)
12 months: 10.2 kg (22 lb 8 oz)

Girls
9 months: 8.6 kg (18 lb 15 oz)
12 months: 9.5 kg (20 lb 5 oz)
Weight tripled in first year
Weight gain 100 g (3½ oz) per week

AVERAGE LENGTH
Boys
9 months: 72.5 cm (28 in)
12 months: 76 cm (30 in)

Girls
9 months: 70 cm (27½ in)
12 months: 74 cm (29 in)
By 12 months length has increased
50 per cent from birth.

DEVELOPMENT
- Can pick up objects
- Babbles
- Dribbling stops
- Sits in high chair for feeding
- Can hold a cup
- Crawls/walks
- Knows name
- Wants to feed self
- At 9 months can learn to drink from cup
- Eight teeth present by 12 months

DIET
- Eats a good variety of food
- Still requires 600–700 ml (21–24 fl oz) breast milk or formula daily
- Takes sandwiches and bread easily.
- Snacks are important
- Sugar, salt, honey and butter/margarine still avoided except for a scraping on bread
- Baby cereals continued (adult cereals too high in salt and fibre and too low in iron)
- Small amounts of whole cow's milk can now be offered in a cup, but not as main milk drink
- Whole eggs can now be given
- Finger foods should be encouraged

TEXTURE AND FEEDING NOTES
- Highly textured — chopped or very roughly mashed
- Without molar teeth, meat may be difficult to chew — still needs to be minced
- Spicy, sugary or fatty foods to be avoided
- Always check temperature of food before serving, especially if using a microwave oven
- For recipe ideas see *Chewable Choices* on page 63

SAMPLE MENU
At 12 months

Breakfast
Breast milk or formula
Cereal with milk
Toast

AM
Diluted juice
Piece of fruit

Lunch
Sandwich
Fruit
Milk, breast milk or formula

PM
Diluted juice

Dinner
Small serve meat, chicken or fish
Egg
Vegetables
Custard
Milk

Before bed
Breast milk or formula (if needed)

Ages and Stages: 1 to 3 years

AVERAGE WEIGHT

Boys
12 months: 10.2 kg (22 lb 8 oz)
3 years: 14.2 kg (32 lb 8 oz)

Girls
12 months: 9.5 kg (20 lb 15 oz)
3 years: 13.9 kg (31 lb)
Weight gain about 2 kg (4.4 lb) per year

AVERAGE LENGTH

Boys:
12 months: 76 cm (30 in)
3 years: 96.5 cm (38 in)

Girls:
12 months: 74 cm (29 in)
3 years: 95.5 cm (37 in)
Length increases 12 cm (5 in)/year at 1–2 years and 9 cm (4 in)/year at 2–3 years

DEVELOPMENT

- Drinks from a cup
- Can kick a ball
- Builds a tower
- Jumps on spot
- Talkative by 18 months
- Walks alone
- By two, puts two words together
- Toilet training underway
- Explores, climbs, gets into mischief
- Imaginative play
- Draws circles
- Likes nursery rhymes
- Toddler stage begins about 12 to 18 months
- Independent, has definite likes and dislikes, short memory
- Everything must be done now!
- Proportions of body change — legs are long and thin; protruding stomach disappears
- Feeds himself
- Full set of 20 teeth

DIET

- Growth has slowed down, so appetite smaller. May need to eat six small meals daily rather than three large ones
- Eats family diet with varied foods
- Milk still important — 600 ml (21 fl oz) daily (whole, not reduced or low fat)
- Can use cow's milk from 12 months, instead of breast milk or formula
- Encouraging fruits, vegetables, breads and cereals and water helps to avoid constipation
- Too much juice can cause diarrhoea
- Fussy eating/food fads may begin
- Child will develop firm likes and dislikes
- Encourage water when thirsty

TEXTURE AND FEEDING NOTES

- Texture and food as for whole family
- Remember:
  – A child only eats if he is hungry
  – A child who refuses food is not hungry
  – No healthy child ever starved from refusing food. See Chapter 4
- See page 67 for recipe ideas

SAMPLE MENU
At 3 years

Breakfast
Cereal
Toast
Milk

AM
Piece fruit
Milk

Lunch
Sandwich
Milk

PM
1 slice bread
Diluted juice

Dinner
Small serve meat
1 serve potato and vegetables
Custard
Fruit
Water

Ages and Stages: 3 to 5 years

AVERAGE WEIGHT
Boys
3 years: 14.7 kg (32 lb 8 oz)
5 years: 18.5 kg (41 lb)

Girls
3 years: 13.9 kg (31 lb)
5 years: 17.8 kg (39 lb 8 oz)
Average weight gain 2 kg (4.4 lb) per year

AVERAGE LENGTH
Boys
3 years: 96.5 cm (38 in)
5 years: 110 cm (44 in)

Girls
3 years: 95.5 cm (37 in)
5 years: 108 cm (43 in)
Birth length has doubled by 4 years
Average length increase 7 cm (3 in)/year

DEVELOPMENT
- Tries to help
- Becomes cooperative
- Language well developed
- Very physical actions
- Can be reasoned with
- Dresses himself
- Quite independent
- Applies what he has learnt to everyday tasks
- Copies
- Teething finished — second teeth come at 6 years
- Sits at family table
- Ready to learn table manners
- Interested in own body and how it works

DIET
- Family foods
- Should avoid too much sugar, fat and salts, 'junk foods'
- Healthy snack foods provided
- Acquires new taste for different foods
- Can still be fussy
- Continues on whole milk until at least 5 years
- Water to be encouraged

TEXTURE AND FEEDING NOTES
- Snacks are important
- Child can be encouraged to help with food preparation and to set table
- Forcing a child to eat a food he doesn't like will never make him like it
- For recipe ideas see *Kindergarten Kids* on page 69

SAMPLE MENU
At 5 years

Breakfast
Juice or fruit
Cereal
Toast

AM
Fruit

Lunch
Sandwich
Fruit
Milk

PM
Cheese sticks
Slice of bread

Dinner
Small serve meat
1 serve potato and vegetables
Fruit
Milk

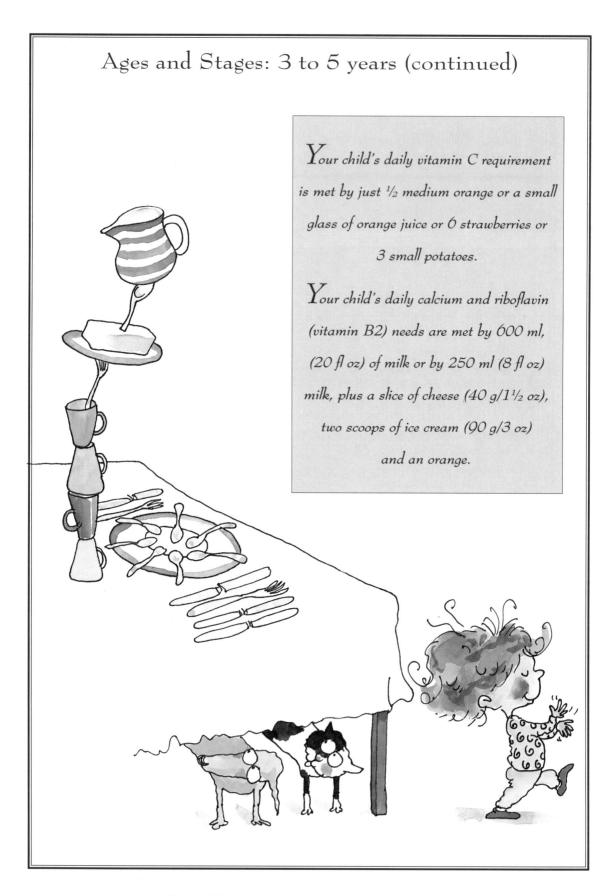

*Y*our child's daily vitamin C requirement is met by just ½ medium orange or a small glass of orange juice or 6 strawberries or 3 small potatoes.

*Y*our child's daily calcium and riboflavin (vitamin B2) needs are met by 600 ml, (20 fl oz) of milk or by 250 ml (8 fl oz) milk, plus a slice of cheese (40 g/1½ oz), two scoops of ice cream (90 g/3 oz) and an orange.

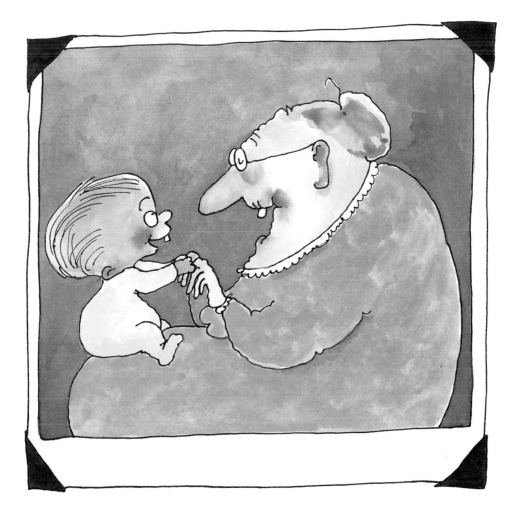

Ouch! Another tooth

Most babies can chew very well without teeth, so don't keep your baby on puréed food just because he doesn't have any — many a toothless baby has 'eaten' a biscuit with great relish!

Occasionally, babies are born with a tooth (apparently Julius Caesar was such a baby). Such a tooth will usually be removed in case the baby swallows it. More commonly the first tooth is cut somewhere between 6 and 7 months. This is usually one of the lower central incisors (or 'front bottom', in parent-speak!), followed by the one next to it. The top teeth usually follow. Some babies 'cross cut', so that the bottom tooth cut doesn't correspond with the top tooth, but it doesn't seem to bother the baby!

These first little teeth are designed for biting off foods, while chewing is always done at the back of the mouth. Even without back teeth, gums are tough and your baby will be able to chew quite lumpy foods by 6 months.

By 12–15 months the first molar appears, making chewing considerably easier. The canines or 'eye teeth' usually come through at around 18 months and some time after the second birthday, the second molars or 'two-year-old teeth' appear.

During all of this teething business, foods which can be chewed are very desirable and must be encouraged. Teething toys and hard rusks are also important for gum and jaw exercise. Always take care that your baby is never left alone while eating. He can easily bite off a big chunk of food but then not have enough teeth to chew it properly, so that it can catch in his throat and cause him to choke. By being with him, you allow him to chew on everything.

A teething baby is always a concern to parents. Your baby may whinge, dribble a lot and have very flushed cheeks. When you've done everything you can and he's still unhappy, you put it down to the fact that he is teething.

Unfortunately many illnesses are misdiagnosed as teething problems when in fact medical attention is needed. If you are not sure and your baby is unwell, always check with your doctor — don't just assume it is a teething problem, because it may not be.

Caring for teeth

Tooth decay is very nasty and not uncommon in young children. Once teeth appear, you can clean them by gently rubbing with a piece of cotton material. Buy your baby a very soft baby toothbrush and give it to him in his bath: instinctively he will put it straight into his mouth!

As he gets a little older and has more teeth, show him how to gently brush. A tiny dot of toothpaste, while not necessary, will be 'required' when he sees you using it.

Nutrition is very important in the care of teeth. Protein and calcium are important for the health of your baby's teeth, and fluoride is important when teeth are developing. If you live in an area where water is not fluoridated, you may need to give your baby fluoride drops. If you are not sure, check with your dentist.

Foods such as breast milk, formula, cow's milk and fruit juices can cause your baby's teeth to decay if allowed to sit around the teeth for a period of time. This situation may occur if your baby falls asleep at the breast or with a bottle in his mouth. A good rule of thumb for healthy teeth is to always offer fluids other than formula or breast milk in a cup — the fluid is swallowed rather than left sitting in the mouth.

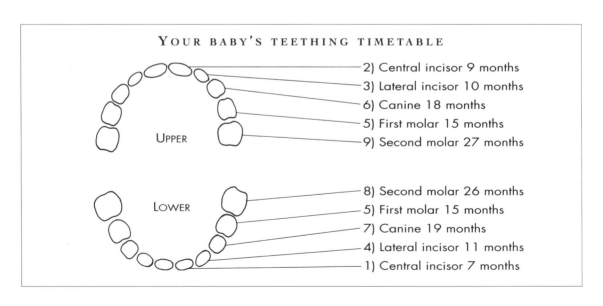

YOUR BABY'S TEETHING TIMETABLE

UPPER
- 2) Central incisor 9 months
- 3) Lateral incisor 10 months
- 6) Canine 18 months
- 5) First molar 15 months
- 9) Second molar 27 months

LOWER
- 8) Second molar 26 months
- 5) First molar 15 months
- 7) Canine 19 months
- 4) Lateral incisor 11 months
- 1) Central incisor 7 months

CHAPTER FOUR

HELP! MY CHILD WON'T EAT

The pressing question of quantity

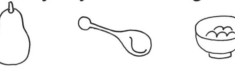

How much is enough?

Children have a simple yet perfect appetite control mechanism — they eat when they're hungry and drink when they're thirsty. By the time we're adults we seem to have grown out of this inbuilt ability to stop when we've had enough, so we easily become obsessed with the question of whether our children are eating enough; having children with a 'healthy appetite' is very closely connected with our image of good parenting.

Concern about a child's appetite is especially prevalent after 12 months of age. In just a few months we have watched our babies progress from half a teaspoon of rice cereal to three square (if down-sized) meals a day. Without giving it too much thought, we seem to expect their appetites to keep growing at the same rate.

But as we've seen from the last chapter, their bodies don't keep growing at the same rate — if they did, our babies would all be giants by the time they went to school! Look again at these facts taken from the *Ages and Stages* tables on pages 43–50.

• In the first year of a baby's life he triples his weight, gaining some 7 kg (15 lb). From then on he gains only 2 kg (4.4 lb) per year.

• In the first year a baby's height increases by 50 per cent or about 25 cm (10 in). From age 1–2 years, height increases by only 12 cm (5 in) and from 2–3 years by just 8 cm (3 in). Around this time your baby will use up his 'baby fat' from his tummy, legs and arms as his bones lengthen, and muscles will firm up and strengthen.

As your baby grows older, energy is needed more for activity and less for growth. Between 6 and 12 months, 6 per cent of energy is needed for growth and 14 per cent for activity. From 2–5 years, only 2 per cent of energy is needed for growth while 23–28 per cent is needed for activity. (The rest is required for maintenance of body functions.)

Unfortunately, unrealistic expectations about how much a child should eat can lead you to think you have a small or fussy eater or a food refuser sitting in that highchair, and your efforts to solve a problem that doesn't yet exist could actually create it.

Consider how off-putting *you* find it to be served too much food on a plate. Children feel the same. They might refuse food not because they don't like it but because it just looks too much for their little stomachs to handle. And when they are told that they must finish everything on the plate before they can leave the table — well, it all becomes a bit too much and rejection, stubbornness and tantrums set in, making the mealtime a disaster.

Serve young children small portions and if they're still hungry they can ask for more. Three small meals and two snacks daily suits most children much better than three large meals.

Just as adults vary their food intake from day to day, so will children, so don't

Food Group	Serving size	Number of Serves				
		1 year	2 years	3 years	4 years	5 years
Bread and cereals	1 slice bread ½ bread roll 2 plain savoury biscuits ½–1 cup (30 g/1 oz) cereal ½ cup (130 g/4½ oz) cooked porridge 1 wheat flake biscuit ½ cup (90 g/3 oz) cooked pasta or rice	4	4	5	5	5
Fruit and vegetables	1 piece fruit 125 ml (4 fl oz) fruit juice (110 g/4 oz) 'toddler' fruit ¼ cup (35 g/1 oz) cooked vegetables ½ potato ½ carrot	3	4	4	4	4
Dairy foods	200 ml (6½ fl oz) milk 200 g (6½ oz) yoghurt 40 g (1½ oz) cheese 200 ml (6½ fl oz) custard	3	3	3	3	3
Meat and substitutes	30 g (1 oz) lean meat, fish, poultry 1 egg 1 tablespoon peanut butter ½ cup (140 g/5 oz) baked beans 1 fish finger	1	2	2	2	2
Fats and oils	2 teaspoons	1	1	2	2	2

APPROXIMATE DAILY NEEDS FOR CHILDREN 1 TO 5 YEARS

always expect your child to eat as much today as he did yesterday. Look at the balance of nutrients taken over a week not just one day: what is missed one day will often be picked up the next.

If you take another look at the *Ages and Stages* tables in the last chapter, you'll notice from the sample menus that a 5-year-old eats roughly the same as a 1-year-old. On the opposite page is another table showing in more detail what it's reasonable to expect your child to eat over the same span of ages. Naturally this will vary according to how active your child is and whether he is going through a growth spurt, but notice how little the amount of food increases overall.

Can't you eat more than that?

*R*obbie's an energetic, busy 2-year-old, but just won't eat anything. He can't sit down long enough to eat and only fiddles and picks at his food. I'm afraid he's going to fade away to a shadow.

Does this sound familiar? To most of us with children between 18 months and 4 years, the answer will be a definite 'yes'. It's one thing to congratulate ourselves on not having unreasonable expectations about how much a child will eat, but quite another to stand by and watch him eat virtually nothing for days.

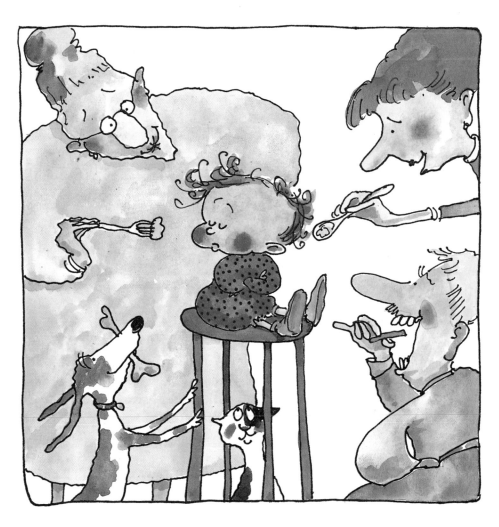

Many young children have quite adult tastes — they like olives, pâté, strong cheeses, spicy foods, pizza, and mild curries and Chinese foods. Let them try these.

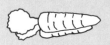

Your child's daily iron requirement can be met by an egg plus a thin slice of beef (30 g/1 oz), a serve of cereal and 4 slices of bread.

The first and most important thing to remember is this:

No healthy child ever starved through refusing food.
When your child is hungry enough, he will eat.

You will also find it comforting to remember that periods of food refusal are actually quite normal, especially for toddlers. Toddlers are wilful little creatures who are just beginning to savour the satisfaction of manipulating those big people who, all their lives, have been telling them what to do.

They soon learn that saying 'no' to food provokes a much better reaction than saying 'no' to playing with their blocks or to patting the dog, even if they don't understand why you invest more emotion in the food.

However, food refusal is not always attributable to contrariness. You will probably recognise when your child is just trying to 'push your button' for a reaction. If you don't feel this is the cause, it's a good idea to ask yourself these questions:

• What has your child eaten through the day? Has he eaten too many snacks? Drunk too much milk or fruit juice? Too much milk or fruit juice will easily take the edge off a child's appetite. Two cups of orange juice are equivalent to four oranges!

• Is this the normal time for meals or is it earlier or later?

• Is your child upset, tired, teething, cranky, or sick? No child wants to eat if he feels like this.

• Does he like the food being served? Have you given him too much on his plate? Does the food look attractive?

• Has there been a change in the family situation that might threaten your child's security?

• Has he got the right chair and his own utensils for eating?

• Has he been less active than usual during the day?

Even if you can find a probable cause, ongoing food refusal can be difficult to cope with. Many parents find it very stressful to see their children eating very little, not to mention the frustration of preparing meals only to have them pushed away.

If you are concerned, keep a food diary for several days, writing down everything your child eats and drinks. Check your lists against the quantities suggested on page 54; if you feel your child really isn't getting enough, have a chat with your doctor, dietitian or baby health nurse. They can measure and weigh your child and either reassure you that he is growing at the right rate for his age or, if necessary, recommend some measures to get him back on track.

There are milk powders formulated for children who do not eat well. These have added vitamins and minerals and contain minimal sugar and no artificial colours or flavours; they may be of help if you're concerned. If your child requires a vitamin or mineral supplement, take care to choose one recommended for children. Such supplements should only be used on the advice of your doctor or dietitian.

MANAGING FOOD REFUSAL

Nobody says that managing food refusal is a breeze, but you can make it easier on yourself by following these tips:

• Ensure your child is hungry before mealtimes. Fresh air, exercise and sleep help stimulate good appetites — make sure your child is getting plenty of each.

• Make mealtimes sociable, happy occasions and keep the atmosphere peaceful. Avoid eating in front of the TV, while the radio is on or while reading, and don't play games while eating. Make sure your child sits down to eat, as eating on the run can be dangerous.

• Use suitable feeding equipment — fork, spoon, plate, cup. Let your child go with you to buy his feeding equipment. Provide a bib, especially for the messy eater. A highchair or small table and chair are essential.

• Children are creatures of habit and routine. Make sure meals and snacks are at regular times throughout the day.

• Don't get cross with a child if he doesn't eat. If anger is associated with meals, he will be even less inclined to eat. And donot prolong the mealtime. If your child refuses to eat, quietly remove the food and allow him to leave the table.

• If your child has refused a meal, avoid offering substitute foods. Wait until the next scheduled meal or snack.

• Never insist that a child finishes everything on his plate. Remember, children know when they have had enough.

• Let children select the foods they want from what is offered. This makes them feel grown-up.

• Don't worry about mess and spills. Cover the floor under the highchair and table with an old sheet or plastic tablecloth so that mess is easily cleaned up.

• Encourage meals with the family where possible and practical — this is a special treat for most toddlers.

• Let your child help with food preparation. He can watch as you prepare vegetables, let him add herbs and spices to sauces and taste them for flavour. Most children from age 3 can help with measuring, pouring, stirring, kneading, decorating and arranging food on a plate. Children love to prepare sandwiches, make simple pizzas and peel their own bananas. Talk about the food as you prepare it.

• Encourage your child to try new foods. This is made easier by letting him help prepare them when possible. New foods are best introduced when a child is hungry. Show your pleasure when he eats and likes a new food.

• Don't influence your child into your own likes and dislikes. Set an example by eating the same food without commenting that you may not like it.

• Don't bribe with special foods or dessert. This only makes these foods more 'special' than other foods.

• Stick to one-course meals and only offer desserts on special occasions. If the child refuses the food offered, accept that the meal is over.

Fussy, Fussy, Fussy

MY CHILD WON'T DRINK MILK

Many children prefer it flavoured. Serve it as milk shakes, custard, use in soups, make white sauces, add to vegetables. Yoghurt and cheese are excellent substitutes for milk (see table on page 54). If your child doesn't enjoy cow's milk, try a soy milk that has added vitamins and minerals. If no dairy products are taken, your child may need a calcium supplement, see your doctor or dietitian.

MY CHILD WON'T DRINK WATER

This is very common but it is important to encourage water intake. Serve it cold from the fridge — it tastes better this way — or as ice blocks, or try a water purifier. If your child won't drink plain water, try flavouring it with a slice of lemon, or use part of the daily fruit juice allowance and dilute with water. Cordial can also be used diluted 1:20.

MY CHILD WON'T EAT VEGETABLES

Often children who will not eat cooked vegetables will enjoy them raw or blanched as a snack. Use celery, carrot and salad vegetables. Fruits have the same nutrients as vegetables so are an excellent substitute. Small amounts of fruit and vegetable juices can also be given (restrict to 1–2 drinks per day).

MY CHILD WON'T EAT MEAT

Many people feel that a meal is not a meal without meat: this is not true. The protein and iron in meat can also be found in wholegrain cereals and bread, eggs, milk products, legumes and ground nuts. Children love peanut butter and baked beans which are both good substitutes for meat (see table on page 54). Many children don't eat meat because they are unable to chew it properly until the second molars come through after 2 years. Serve meat soft, minced or finely chopped with gravy if your child has difficulty eating it — savoury minces and casseroles are usually well-liked.

MY CHILD ONLY EATS WHITE BREAD

White bread is a nutritious food containing protein, complex carbohydrate, fibre, vitamins and minerals, although the quantities of nutrients are lower than in wholemeal bread. For extra fibre (the same as in wholemeal), use the white high fibre loaves. Encourage your child to eat a variety of breads, but remember that many children do not like the grains in mixed grain breads nor the colour or texture of wholemeal breads. White bread is better than no bread.

MY CHILD WON'T EAT ANY OF THE FOOD I PREPARE

Your child is going through a very common food fad stage. Prepare foods you know your child likes. Check that you are not overcooking vegetables and meat, that food looks attractive and serving sizes are not too big. Try wrapping sandwiches and putting them in a bag so your child thinks they are bought. Put the custard you have made in a washed yoghurt container. Try commercial children's cuisine — excellent in nutrition, flavour and texture for children 18 months to 5 years and a great, cheap substitute when children go through this phase. Or use commercial foods as a base and add your own extras.

Fussy, Fussy, Fussy

MY CHILD WON'T EAT ANYTHING BUT CHEESE SANDWICHES

Again, another common stage. Go along with it without fuss. It will pass in time. Cheese sandwiches are still nutritious!

MY CHILD EATS TOO MUCH AFTERNOON TEA AND THEN WON'T EAT DINNER

Most children seem to be ravenous at about 3.30–4.00 pm. If practical, serve the main course of dinner at this time, and then a snack, drink or dessert at dinner time. It is important that your child does not fill up on non-nutritious foods such as lollies, cakes, biscuits or chips at this time.

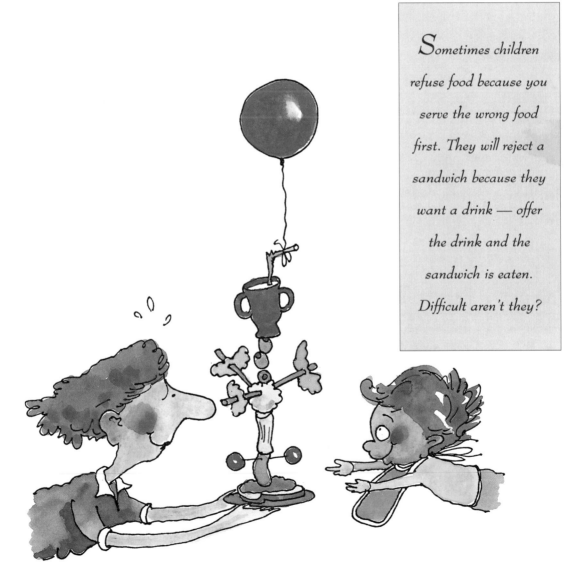

Sometimes children refuse food because you serve the wrong food first. They will reject a sandwich because they want a drink — offer the drink and the sandwich is eaten. Difficult aren't they?

~

CHAPTER FIVE

So, What's for Dinner?

Our easy, nutritious recipes

A NOTE ABOUT SERVING SIZES

You will notice in *First Foods* and *More Tastes and Textures* that in most cases we have not specified how many servings our recipes will make. This is because, as we have discussed at some length, the amount a child eats today will be different to the amount he ate yesterday, so we felt that including serving numbers would only cause confusion and sometimes even anxiety. You will easily see from the quantity of ingredients whether your child is likely to eat the whole lot at one sitting or whether you will have extra servings left over for freezing.

FIRST FOODS *(4 to 6 months)*

FRUIT PURÉE

Apples or pears

Wash and peel carefully. Cut into pieces. Microwave or steam until soft. Fork mash, adding cooled boiled water or formula until you get the right consistency.

Commercial baby foods also provide an excellent range of fruits, select those prepared without added sugar.

~

MEAT PURÉE

PREPARATION TIME: 5 MINUTES
FREEZING: SUITABLE

Steamed, diced breast of chicken without skin, or piece of tender roast beef, or tender meat from stew

You need a food processor to really blend meat smoothly. Add a little boiled water or gravy until purée is the consistency of thick gravy. Serve ½–1 teaspoon and freeze the remainder in an ice cube tray.

Babies prefer moist foods.

~

Perfect Vegetable Purée

SAVE TIME BY PREPARING AT THE
FAMILY MEAL TIME.
FREEZING: SUITABLE

1 piece pumpkin or potato

Wash and peel carefully. Cut into pieces. Microwave or steam until soft. Fork mash, adding cooled boiled water or formula until you get the right consistency.

At first, most babies refuse any food which may have the slightest hint of a lump. The high water content in potato and pumpkin means you can get a perfect purée by just continuing to mash with a fork. Babies do not like the 'claggy' feel of potato that is too thick, so thin down to a sloppy consistency at first.

~

Fish Purée

PREPARATION TIME: 10 MINUTES
FREEZING: SUITABLE

1 fillet of fish
2 tablespoons mashed potato

Steam fish until tender. Purée in food processor. Add mashed potato. Thin with a little boiled water. Serve ½–1 teaspoon at first and freeze the remainder in small portions in an ice cube tray.

~

Apple Rice

1 tablespoon infant rice cereal
1 tablespoon apple purée
apple juice (optional)

Mix cereal and apple, then mix with apple juice to a 'sloppy' consistency. Place 1–2 tablespoons in baby's serving bowl, then place remainder in a small airtight container and refrigerate. (This will thicken in fridge. Thin with a little extra juice or water before serving.)

VARIATION: Substitute pear, apricot or banana purée for apple purée.

Use commercial fruit purées, with no added sugar, if you only need small quantities.

~

MORE TASTES AND TEXTURES *(6 to 9 months)*

Creamy Rice with Banana

PREPARATION TIME: 5 MINUTES
FREEZING: NOT SUITABLE

1 tablespoon cooked rice
1 tablespoon whole milk yoghurt
½ large or 1 small banana
cinnamon (optional)

Mash banana into small lumps. Mix with yoghurt and cooked rice. Place half the quantity in baby's serving bowl and refrigerate the remainder in a small airtight container for up to 48 hours.

VARIATION: Substitute puréed pears or apples for banana. Try adding cinnamon.

~

GREEN FINGERS

PREPARATION TIME: 5 MINUTES
FREEZING: NOT SUITABLE

2 teaspoons mashed ripe avocado
1 slice thick toasting bread

Toast bread and allow to cool. Spread with mashed avocado. Cut into three fingers. Offer one finger at a time.

A delicious snack for mum too!

~

VEGETABLE CHIPS

PREPARATION TIME: 5 MINUTES
FREEZING: SUITABLE

small pieces carrot, celery and potato

Cut into straws. Steam or microwave until tender. Cool, then offer 1–2 of each. Store remainder in an airtight container in the fridge.

~

ROUGH VEGETABLES

PREPARATION TIME: 5 MINUTES
FREEZING: SUITABLE

small pieces (about 4 cm/1 ½ in) carrot, parsnip and potato, plus a few peas

Prepare vegetables, steam or microwave until tender, use a coarse attachment on the baby mouli or fork mash roughly for more texture. If too textured, add a little cool boiled water or formula.

A food processor tends to process baby's food too fine now — and it is awful to wash! — so once baby can manage more textured foods, don't bother with it.

~

CHICKEN SUPREME

PREPARATION TIME: 5 MINUTES
FREEZING: NOT SUITABLE

1 tablespoon minced chicken
1 tablespoon mashed potato
1 chopped cooked egg yolk
½ tablespoon cooked peas

Combine all ingredients. Add cool boiled water or formula to thin down to a creamy consistency. Offer 1–2 tablespoons and place the remainder in a small airtight container in the fridge.

Only egg yolk should be used, as egg white may cause an allergy. Wait until your baby is about 9 months before trying egg white. Leftover egg whites can be chopped up and added to sandwich fillings for the rest of the family.

~

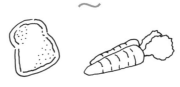

RUSKS

PREPARATION TIME: 2 MINUTES

4 slices thick toasting bread

Trim off crusts, cut each slice into three fingers and bake in slow oven for one hour.

Commercial rusks are excellent and save a lot of time and bother, but make sure you use the ones with no added sugar. Rusks are not really meant to be eaten but are to bite or chew on. Babies will enjoy rusks plain — there is no need to add yeast extracts, honey or jam. The latter contain sugar which may damage his teeth. Serve one at a time. Store in an airtight container.

~

CHEWABLE CHOICES *(9 to 12 months)*

MUESLI WITH FRUIT

PREPARATION TIME: 2 MINUTES

2 tablespoons infant muesli
60 g (2 oz) canned or bottled commercial baby
fruit (e.g. peach, apple, apricot), with no added
sugar
Formula or boiled cow's milk

Add fruit to muesli, and enough milk
to give a 'soggy' consistency. Do not
keep leftovers.

*Always add warmed milk to cereal and fruit,
never microwave milk, cereal and fruit
together — there is a danger of hot spots
and a scalded mouth.*

~

LITTLE MEATBALLS

PREPARATION TIME: 5 MINUTES
FREEZING: SUITABLE

250 g (8 oz) lean minced steak
½ onion finely chopped
1 tablespoon soy sauce
½ teaspoon sugar
½ teaspoon powdered ginger
1 teaspoon oil

Combine all ingredients. Make
meatballs using a teaspoon of mixture.
Paint a heavy bottomed frypan with
cooking oil, or use a non-stick pan (in
which case no oil is needed). Heat and cook
quickly until brown. Serve a few meatballs
warm or cold. Freeze the remainder.

MAKES 8–10

*This is a good recipe for
party food as well
as for everyday fare.*

~

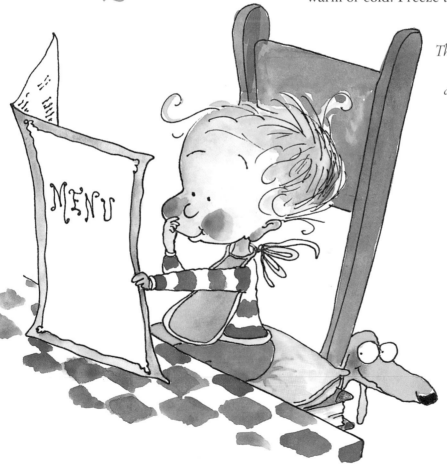

Fish Balls

PREPARATION TIME: 15 MINUTES
FREEZING: SUITABLE
MAKES 10–12

2 large potatoes
½ onion
180 g (6 oz) canned tuna (salt reduced)
½ carrot, grated
1 small zucchini (courgette), grated
1 egg
plain (all-purpose) flour

Peel potato and onion and cut into chunks. Cook until soft, then mash until smooth. (Do not use food processor as potato 'overprocesses' and will go very watery.) Add remaining ingredients except flour. Shape into balls, roll in flour and cook quickly in a lightly greased frypan or a non-stick pan. Delicious warm or cold. Serve with snow peas, shredded lettuce and tomato slices.

Noodles with Cheese

PREPARATION TIME: 10 MINUTES
FREEZING: NOT SUITABLE

¼ cup (40 g/1½ oz) noodles
½ tomato, finely diced
1 tablespoon sweet corn kernels
1 tablespoon grated cheese
1 tablespoon smooth ricotta
chopped fresh parsley

Cook noodles. Combine all ingredients and sprinkle with chopped parsley. Serve 1–2 tablespoons to your baby as a meal. For the rest of the family, serve as an accompaniment to meat.

~

Fried Rice

PREPARATION TIME: 15 MINUTES
FREEZING: NOT SUITABLE

½ cup (40 g/1½ oz) white rice
¼ onion, chopped
½ carrot, diced
30 g (1 oz) peas
1 teaspoon oil
1 egg
1 teaspoon soy sauce

Cook rice, onion, carrot and peas and mix together. Beat egg and cook quickly in a lightly oiled frypan. Chop into pieces. Add rice and vegetables, sprinkle with a little soy sauce. Great for lunch or to serve at dinner time with some chopped, cooked chicken pieces. Should be some left over for mum, too!

~

Tasty Meatloaf

PREPARATION TIME: 20 MINUTES
FREEZING: SUITABLE

1 slice bread
2 tablespoons milk
1 clove garlic, crushed
(or 1 teaspoon minced garlic)
1 onion
½ large carrot
1 large cooking apple
500 g (1 lb) lean minced steak
1 tablespoon fruit chutney
1 tablespoon tomato sauce
1 teaspoon mixed herbs
1 egg
dried breadcrumbs

Soak bread in milk. Peel and grate onion, carrot and apple. Combine all ingredients and mix thoroughly. Shape into a loaf, sprinkle breadcrumbs on top, wrap in foil and bake on a tray in a moderate oven 50–60 minutes. Open up top of foil and continue cooking a further 10–15 minutes. Serve hot with mashed potatoes, carrot rings and beans. Serves 4 adults. Also delicious cold as a sandwich filling or with salad.

VARIATION: Use any combination of vegetables you have at hand — peas, corn, potato and tomato are tasty additions.

~

BEANS ON RYE

PREPARATION TIME: 2 MINUTES

2 slices rye bread
125 g (4 oz) canned baked beans (salt reduced)

Toast rye bread. Mash baked beans and spread on toast. Cut into three fingers, then cut each finger in half. Serve 2–3 squares at a time.

Rye bread makes a delicious change to wholemeal and white bread. Offer light rye bread at first. If your baby enjoys it, try the darker, heavier rye another time. A great lunch for mum, too!

~

BASIC WHITE SAUCE

PREPARATION TIME: 15 MINUTES
FREEZING: SUITABLE

2 cups (500 ml/16 fl oz) milk
2 tablespoons cornflour

Bring milk to the boil, mix cornflour to a thin paste with a little cold water and add to milk. Stir until thickens.

Use this as a basis for easy recipes — add grated cheese, chopped chives or parsley for variety. Add a tablespoon of sugar to the cornflour for a sweet white sauce — delicious served hot or cold with fruit.

~

CHICKEN EASY

PREPARATION TIME: 30 MINUTES
FREEZING: SUITABLE

½ cup (90 g/3 oz) noodles
½ onion
1 carrot
½ parsnip
1 quantity Basic White Sauce
500 g (1 lb) chicken, diced and cooked
2 tablespoons grated cheese

Cook noodles. Cut onion, carrot and parsnip into 1 cm (½ in) dice and cook. Combine all ingredients and place in casserole dish. Cook at 200°C (400°F) for ½ hour to warm through. Serves 4 adults.

~

APRICOT CRUMBLE

PREPARATION TIME: 10 MINUTES
FREEZING: SUITABLE

440 g (14 oz) canned 'pie-pack' apricots (solid fruit without syrup)
1 teaspoon cinnamon
2 cups (200 g/7 oz) infant muesli

Place apricots in a lightly greased pie dish and cover with muesli, then sprinkle with cinnamon. Warm through 10 minutes at 200°C (400°F). Serve with custard. Delicious for the whole family. Serves 4 adults.

Packet custard powder is a quick and convenient way to make custard. If your baby has a milk-free formula, simply substitute his formula for cow's milk to make milk-free custard.

~

Finger Foods

Chewing is very important for your baby's tooth and jaw development. When he feels a bit 'peckish', offer a suitable nutritious finger food which will encourage him to chew.

FRUIT AND VEGETABLE STICKS

Slice fruit such as pear, banana and orange (with the pith removed), and offer one or two pieces at a time.

Cut vegetables such as potato, carrot, celery and French beans into straws and lightly steam to soften. Keep a small supply in the fridge and offer two or three pieces at a time.

~

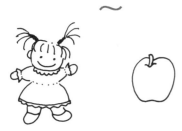

BREAD FINGERS

Thick slices of toast cut into fingers and lightly spread with peanut butter, mashed avocado, cheddar cheese spread, yeast extract or ricotta cheese are always popular.

~

CRACKERS WITH CREAM CHEESE

Spread cream cheese thickly on a plain cracker. Your baby will love licking it off then crunching on the cracker.

~

MINI SANDWICHES

Make a sandwich with a favourite filling, trim off crusts and cut into an interesting shape with a fancy biscuit cutter. Otherwise cut into triangles and then cut each triangle again. Babies delight in small morsels of food!

~

CHICKEN CHIPS

Steam a chicken breast, allow to cool then cut into strips. Sometimes meat on its own is a bit dry so place some plain yoghurt on your baby's plate and show him how to dip the chicken pieces into the yoghurt. He will love eating the yoghurt with his fingers, too!

~

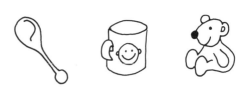

Temptations for Toddlers (1 to 3 years)

Many young children have quite 'gourmet' tastes and enjoy foods such as pickled onions, gherkins, pâté and mild curries. Children are generally quite adventurous, particularly if you are. Many of these recipes will also be enjoyed by mum and dad!

Penny's Paté

PREPARATION TIME: 5 MINUTES
FREEZING: SUITABLE

250 g (8 oz) liverwurst spread
grated rind and juice of one orange
¼ bunch fresh parsley, chopped
black pepper (optional)

Mix ingredients together, press into a small bowl. Refrigerate for ½ hour before serving. Spread on toast fingers or crackers.

For mum and dad, add 3 tablespoons of port instead of the orange!

~

Crusty Topped Savoury Mince

PREPARATION TIME: 15 MINUTES
FREEZING: SUITABLE

500 g (1 lb) minced beef
1–2 teaspoons curry powder
1 onion, chopped
1 green apple, chopped
1 carrot, diced
2 cups (500 ml/16 fl oz) water
1 tablespoon Worcestershire sauce
1 tablespoon cornflour
2 slices bread, crusts removed and cut
into 1 cm (½ in) dice

Brown meat, curry powder and onion in a heavy-bottomed saucepan. Add apple, carrot, water and Worcestershire sauce, cover and simmer ½ hour. Mix cornflour with a little water to make a paste. Add to mixture, boil until thickened. Pour into casserole. Place bread cubes on top. Bake in 200°C (400°F) oven for 45 minutes. Mashed potato can be used in place of bread cubes. Serves 4 adults.

~

Gourmet Lunch

PREPARATION TIME: 5 MINUTES

1–2 cocktail onions
1 cherry tomato
1–2 cubes or sticks of cheese
2 crackers with Penny's Pâté
tuft of alfalfa sprouts

This is a tasty lunch that's easy to prepare. Cut the onions and tomato in half. Arrange on a small plate with cheese and crackers, then add sprouts.

~

Pizza Wheels

PREPARATION TIME: 10 MINUTES
FREEZING: NOT SUITABLE

1 muffin
1 tablespoon grated cheese
½ tomato, diced
1 tablespoon crushed pineapple, drained

Split muffin, pile other ingredients on top and place under griller until cheese melts. Allow to cool, then cut into smaller pieces. Serve with chopped lettuce and carrot straws.

~

CHICKEN WITH APRICOTS

PREPARATION TIME: 15 MINUTES
FREEZING: SUITABLE

4 pieces chicken maryland
1 onion, sliced
1 tablespoon soy sauce
440 g (14 oz) canned pie-pack apricots or
drained canned apricots

Remove skin from chicken, cut each maryland at the joint, and place in casserole dish. Sprinkle with sliced onion and soy sauce. Purée or mash apricots and pour over chicken, cover and cook at 180°C (375°F) for 1½ hours. This is suitable for the whole family. Serves 4 adults.

~

PIKELETS WITH TASTY TOPPINGS

PREPARATION TIME: 30 MINUTES
FREEZING: SUITABLE WHEN COOKED
MAKES 12–18

1 cup (250 g/8 oz) self-raising flour
1 tablespoon sugar
1 egg, lightly beaten
¾ cup (180 ml/6 fl oz) milk

Sift flour, add sugar, add beaten egg and milk. Beat with a wooden spoon until smooth. Heat a heavy bottomed frypan and drop in teaspoons of mixture, 3–4 at a time. Pikelets are cooked when bubbles appear on top. Flip over and cook the other side for a few seconds. Continue until all the mixture is used. Plain pikelets can be frozen.

SUGGESTED TOPPINGS

• Tuna Spread (see recipe below)
• cream cheese with sultanas on top
• cream cheese with sliced banana and a sprinkle of cinnamon
• slice of cheese
• slice of hard-boiled egg
• mashed fruit

VARIATION: Add grated orange or lemon rind to pikelet mixture.

~

TUNA SPREAD

PREPARATION TIME: 15 MINUTES
FREEZING: NOT SUITABLE

220 g (7 oz) canned tuna (salt reduced)
1 tablespoon mayonnaise
1 teaspoon fresh lemon juice
1 teaspoon chopped fresh parsley
½ teaspoon tomato sauce
½ teaspoon Worcestershire sauce
1 teaspoon gelatine dissolved in
1 tablespoon boiling water

Combine all ingredients. Place in a small bowl. Refrigerate until set. Serve on crackers, with salad vegetables or as a sandwich filling.

~

APRICOT YOGHURT DIP

PREPARATION TIME: 10 MINUTES
FREEZING: NOT SUITABLE

6 pieces dried apricots
½ cup (125 ml/4 fl oz) water
¾ cup (200 ml/6 fl oz) vanilla yoghurt
pieces fresh fruit

Soak apricots in water overnight. Blend yoghurt with apricots and any liquid. Serve with pieces of fresh fruit or alone.

This is a great filling for a birthday cake!

~

KINDERGARTEN KIDS *(3 to 5 years)*

You might find your young child now prefers simpler foods compared with his more exotic tastes at 12–18 months. The pre-school years can be very busy and very tiring, so simple food which is easy to eat is best. These recipes will suit your pre-schooler and the whole family. Encourage your child to help you in the kitchen by washing vegetables, placing finger food on plates, mixing, stirring, setting the table and so on.

CORN CHOWDER

PREPARATION TIME: 15 MINUTES
FREEZING: NOT SUITABLE

2 rashers lean bacon
1 large onion
2 large potatoes
1 cup (250 ml/8 fl oz) water
440 g (14 oz) canned creamed corn
1 cup (250 ml/8 fl oz) reduced fat milk

Dice bacon and onion (1 cm/½ in), brown in a little oil in a heavy-bottomed saucepan. Peel and dice potatoes. Add to bacon and onion, stir. Add water. Cover and simmer approximately 20 minutes until potato is cooked. Add creamed corn and milk. Heat through. Do not boil. Serve with crusty bread — great for a quick Sunday lunch. Serves 4 adults.

~

ORANGE SALAD

PREPARATION TIME: 5 MINUTES

snow peas (about 10)
½ large carrot
½ stick celery
1 orange
tuft alfalfa sprouts

Wash snow peas. Cut carrot and celery into fine straws, 3–4 cm (2 in) long. Cut orange in half — peel and dice one half, squeeze juice from the other half. Toss ingredients together. Pour 1 tablespoon orange juice over vegetables. Chill for 1 hour. Serve as an accompaniment to meat. Serves 2–4 adults.

~

SAVOURY RICE

PREPARATION TIME: 15 MINUTES
FREEZING: NOT SUITABLE

1 cup (185 g/6 oz) rice
1 teaspoon oil
500 g (1 lb) lean minced steak
1 clove garlic, crushed
1 onion, chopped
1 cup (250 ml/8 fl oz) water
1 carrot, cut into strips
2 tablespoons soy sauce

Cook rice. Brush oil over the bottom of a large frypan (an electric frypan is good for this recipe). Brown meat with garlic and onion. Add water and carrot. Cover and simmer until vegetables are tender (about 5 minutes). Quickly stir, add cooked rice and soy sauce, stir thoroughly. Serves 4 adults.

~

HIDDEN TREASURES

PREPARATION TIME: 5 MINUTES
FREEZING: NOT SUITABLE

1 pocket bread
1 hard-boiled egg
2 slices tomato
1 teaspoon mayonnaise

Cut pocket bread in half crossways. Slice egg and finely chop lettuce and tomato. Pile ingredients into pocket and drizzle mayonnaise over the top.

VARIATION: Other filling ideas include chopped cold meat with tomato or fruit sauce, grated cheese, tuna with mayonnaise or chopped fresh fruit.

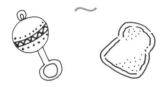

~

EASY SPAGHETTI SAUCE

PREPARATION TIME: 15 MINUTES
FREEZING: SUITABLE

500 g (1 lb) lean minced topside
1 to 2 cloves garlic, crushed
1 onion, chopped
1 teaspoon dried oregano
440 g (14 oz) canned tomato soup (salt reduced)

Brown meat with garlic and onion, add oregano, soup and half a can of water. Stir. Cover and simmer 20 minutes. Serve with cooked spaghetti, or use in lasagne or other pasta dishes. Serves 4 adults.

~

LUNCH TIME FAVOURITES

PREPARATION TIME: 5 MINUTES
FREEZING: NOT SUITABLE

2 slices wholemeal, white or rye bread
margarine
2 tablespoons filling such as:
baked beans
grated cheese
chopped tomato
chopped apple
canned peaches or apricots, drained
sardines, drained
tuna, drained

Switch on snack maker to heat up. Lightly spread bread with margarine then place in snack maker or jaffle iron spread side down. Add filling, place second slice of bread on top with spread side up, close the lid and toast until lightly browned. (If using frypan, follow the same method but turn sandwich over to complete cooking.) Cut into four triangles. Allow to cool. *Take care as the centre of these snacks can become extremely hot.*

~

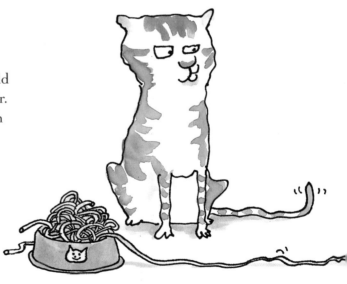

BAKED MACARONI

PREPARATION TIME: 30 MINUTES
FREEZING: SUITABLE

2 cups (90 g/3 oz) macaroni
1 quantity Easy Spaghetti Sauce (see page 70)
6 eggs

Cook macaroni. Lightly grease lasagne dish. Cover with half the macaroni, then meat sauce, then remaining macaroni. Pour beaten eggs over the top. Bake at 200°C (400°F) for 1 hour. Cut into squares. Serves
4 adults. Serve with Orange Salad (see page 69).

~

FRUIT SLAW

¼ cabbage
1 large carrot
½ onion
½ cup drained crushed pineapple
½ cup (90 g/3 oz) sultanas
½ cup (125 ml/4 fl oz) mayonnaise

Shred cabbage, carrot and onion. Place in a large bowl, add remaining ingredients. Chill before serving. Serves 4 adults.

A great way to encourage your child to eat vegetables, you can 'hide' many things this way! This recipe makes a large bowl — keep it refrigerated and add to sandwich fillings or use as a meal accompaniment. Leftovers refrigerated in an airtight container will keep for 48 hours.

~

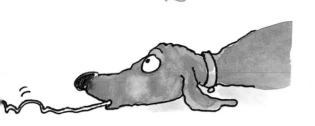

FISH AND CHIPS

PREPARATION TIME: 10 MINUTES
FREEZING: NOT SUITABLE

1 potato per person
1 fish fillet per person
fresh lemon juice

Peel or scrub potatoes and cut into thick chips. Place in a lightly oiled pan and bake for ½ hour at 200°C, turn chips over then continue baking for a further ½ hour. Place fish fillets in pieces in aluminium foil, sprinkle with lemon juice, fold into separate parcels and place in the oven for the last 20 minutes of cooking the chips. Serve with Fruit Slaw.

~

VEGETABLE IDEAS

Some children are not wildly excited about their vegies. However, raw vegetables are often preferred to cooked. Place a platter of raw vegetables on the table and invite your child to choose three colours. Make your platter attractive and always include at least one vegetable you know your child will eat. Try some of the following:

carrot straws
celery sticks
snow peas
green beans (choose young tender ones)
small pieces of cauliflower
small pieces of broccoli

The cauliflower and broccoli can be steamed for 2–3 minutes but served cold. Add pieces of fresh fruit to make it look more exciting, such as a few strawberries, slices of banana or a few grapes. Encourage your child to help you arrange the food on the plate — he may even surprise you by eating some while he's doing it!

~

VEGETARIAN TREATS

You don't have to be vegetarian to enjoy these nutritious and economical dishes for the family.

QUICK VEGETABLE SOUP

PREPARATION TIME: 10 MINUTES
FREEZING: SUITABLE

1 large carrot
1 large onion
1 small parsnip
1 large potato
4 cups (1 litre/32 fl oz) water
4 mixed herb stock cubes
2 tablespoons noodles
¼ bunch parsley, chopped

Peel, wash and grate carrot, onion, parsnip and potato. Combine all ingredients except parsley, simmer for ½ hour. Sprinkle with parsley. Serves 4 adults.

~

VEGETARIAN PARCELS

PREPARATION TIME: 40 MINUTES
FREEZING: SUITABLE WHEN COOKED
MAKES ABOUT 20

1 head broccoli
1 large onion
1 large carrot
½ parsnip
375 g (12 oz) ricotta cheese
¼ teaspoon cinnamon
375 g (12 oz) fillo pastry
1 tablespoon oil
sesame seeds

Cut broccoli into small flowerettes. Discard tough stalks and dice younger, tender stalks. Cut onion, carrot and parsnip into 1 cm (½ in) dice. Microwave or steam until just tender (take care not to overcook). Cool. Add ricotta cheese and cinnamon. Fold out pastry. Take three sheets at a time and cut into four. Prepare all pastry this way and place under a damp cloth to prevent drying out. Place mixture onto pastry, fold in sides and roll into a parcel. Brush with oil and sprinkle with sesame seeds. Place parcels on a lightly greased tray and bake at 200°C (400°F) until lightly brown and crisp.

These are nice hot or cold and great for school lunches.

~

PUMPKIN SOUP

PREPARATION TIME: 30 MINUTES
FREEZING: SUITABLE

500 g (1 lb) pumpkin (after peel and seeds are removed)
1 large onion
1 teaspoon oil
2 mixed herb stock cubes
1 cup (250 ml/8 fl oz) water
2 to 3 peppercorns
1 cup (250 ml/8 fl oz) reduced fat milk

Roughly chop pumpkin and dice (1 cm/½ in) onion. Heat oil in saucepan and gently cook onion without browning. Add pumpkin pieces, crumbled stock cubes, water and peppercorns. Bring to boil, cover and simmer until pumpkin is soft. Allow to cool. Place mixture in blender or mouli and purée. Return to saucepan, add milk and heat through. Serves 4 adults.

~

VEGETARIAN LASAGNE

PREPARATION TIME: 40 MINUTES
FREEZING: SUITABLE

1 large zucchini (courgette)
1 eggplant (aubergine)
1 onion
1 large carrot
1 teaspoon oil
1 clove garlic, crushed
2 tablespoons tomato paste
1 cup (250 ml/8 fl oz) water
220 g (7 oz) 'instant' lasagne
375 g (12 oz) ricotta cheese
1 quantity cheese sauce (see Basic White Sauce
page 65)

Wash zucchini and eggplant, cut into slices, place in colander and lightly sprinkle with salt. Allow to stand ½ hour (this removes the bitterness). Wash and drain well. Slice onion and carrot into rings. Brush oil over the bottom of a large heavy bottomed frypan. Add garlic, onion, carrot, zucchini and eggplant. Brown quickly. Mix tomato paste with water, add to vegetables and simmer gently until tender.

Cool. Lightly brush a lasagne dish with oil. Place a small quantity of vegetable mixture in the bottom, place lasagne noodles on top, cover with more vegetable mixture, half the ricotta cheese, then lasagne. Repeat, finishing with lasagne. Cover with cheese sauce. Bake at 200°C (400°F) for 45 minutes. Serve with crisp salad and crusty bread. Serves 4 adults.

~

BASICALLY EASY BAKING

These recipes can be made for the whole family and are suitable for babies from 9 months old. We have tried to keep added fat to a minimum. You will notice that many other cake and biscuit recipes contain a lot of butter or margarine, often up to 250 g (8 oz). This is all right now and then, but the recipes presented here give you plenty of taste without all the fat. (Commercial biscuits are also high in fat. Don't fall into the trap of dipping into the 'bikkie' barrel every time your baby needs a snack.)

SAVOURY MUFFINS

PREPARATION TIME: 25 MINUTES
FREEZING: SUITABLE
MAKES 12 MUFFINS.

1 cup (125 g/4 oz) self-raising flour
1 cup (125 g/4 oz) self-raising wholemeal flour
1 teaspoon oregano
1 teaspoon chopped fresh parsley
2 tablespoons parmesan cheese
60 g (2 oz) butter
1 cup (250 ml/8 fl oz) milk
1 egg

Sift flours, add herbs and cheese. Melt butter, add milk. Beat egg and add to milk mixture. Stir into flour, but do not overstir — mixture should be a bit lumpy. Spoon into a non-stick muffin tin. Bake at 200°C (400°F) for 35 minutes. Allow to sit 2–3 minutes out of the oven before tipping onto wire cooler.

These freeze very well. Delicious with soup for a weekend lunch.

~

Sweet Muffins

PREPARATION TIME: 25 MINUTES
FREEZING: SUITABLE
MAKES 12 MUFFINS.

1 cup (125 g/4 oz) self-raising flour
1 cup (125 g/4 oz) self-raising wholemeal flour
½ cup (125 g/4 oz) sugar
60 g (2 oz) butter
1 cup (250 ml/8 fl oz) milk
1 egg
1 teaspoon cinnamon
2 green apples, peeled and thinly sliced

Sift flours and add sugar. Melt butter, add milk. Beat egg and add to milk mixture. Stir into flour, but do not overstir — mixture should be a bit lumpy. Stir in cinnamon and apple. Spoon into a non-stick muffin tin. Bake at 200°C (400°F) for 35 minutes. Allow to sit 2–3 minutes out of the oven before tipping onto wire cooler.

Other fruits can be used instead of apples, such as 1 cup (180 g/6 oz) frozen blueberries or 1 cup (240 g/8 oz) pie-pack peaches or apricots.

~

Easy Apple Cake

PREPARATION TIME: 20 MINUTES
FREEZING: SUITABLE

60 g (2 oz) margarine or butter
1 cup (250 g/8 oz) sugar
1½ cups (375 g/12 oz) unsweetened stewed apple or 'pie pack' apple
2 teaspoons bicarbonate of soda
1 teaspoon cinnamon
½ teaspoon nutmeg
1 cup (155 g/5 oz) sultanas
2 cups (250 g/8 oz) plain flour

Cream butter and sugar. Warm apple, stir in soda and add to creamed mixture. Stir in sultanas and fold in sifted flour. Turn into a greased slab tin and bake at 200°C (400°F) for 40–45 minutes. Cut into squares while still warm.

Sultana Cake

PREPARATION TIME: 10 MINUTES
FREEZING: SUITABLE

1 cup (250 ml/8 fl oz) cold strong black tea
1 cup (250 g/8 oz) sugar
1 cup (155 g/5 oz) sultanas
1 cup (125 g/4 oz) self-raising flour
1 egg

Mix tea, sugar and sultanas and allow to soak 2–3 hours. Add beaten egg and sifted flour. Pour into a greased and lined loaf tin. Bake at 200°C (400°F) for 45 minutes.

This is a very moist loaf and is delicious thinly sliced and spread with a little ricotta.

This is a breeze to make, and a good recipe for children to help with.

~

Pastry

PREPARATION TIME: 90 MINUTES
(INCLUDES 1 HOUR RESTING TIME)
FREEZING: SUITABLE TO FREEZE UNCOOKED

It is difficult to make a good pastry with little fat as the result is almost inedible! However, we have come up with a delicious recipe using smooth ricotta cheese. It is very easy to handle and rolls out beautifully. It is suitable for sweet and savoury dishes.

2 cups (250 g/8 oz) plain flour
250 g (8 oz) smooth ricotta cheese
1 egg

Add ricotta to sifted flour and stir evenly. Add lightly beaten egg, and a little cold water (1 to 2 tablespoons) and stir until all the flour is mixed. Tip out on a floured surface and gently knead. Cover in plastic wrap and refrigerate one hour before use.

~

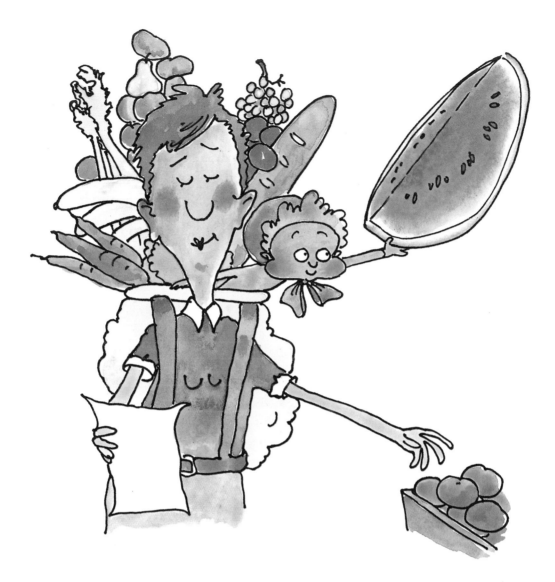

Sweet or Savoury Tartlets

One quantity Pastry (see opposite page)

Suggested fillings

- apple with custard
- pineapple with custard
- sliced banana with yoghurt
- creamed corn
- leftover stew or casserole
- chopped hard-boiled egg with mayonnaise

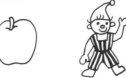

Roll out pastry evenly on a lightly floured surface until 3–4 mm (⅛ in) thick. Cut to required size, using a cutter slightly larger than the tartlet tins. Place pastry rounds in lightly greased tartlet tins, prick with a fork and cook at 220°C (425°F) for 5–10 minutes until golden. Allow to cool, remove from tins and fill.

Store unfilled tartlets in an airtight tin for up to one week. Before use pop into a moderate oven (200°C/400°F) for a few minutes to freshen.

~

BREAD CASES

PREPARATION TIME: 20 MINUTES
FREEZING: SUITABLE (UNFILLED)

12 slices bread
1 egg
1 tablespoon milk

Flatten each slice of bread with a rolling pin. Using a biscuit cutter or large tea cup, cut out the middle of the bread. Beat egg and milk together and brush lightly over bread rounds. Press them into lightly greased patty tins. Bake at 220°C (425°F) for 10 minutes. Bake until crisp and golden. Allow to cool, then fill.

(Cut leftover crusts of bread into pieces and place in the oven to dry out as rusks. Store in an airtight jar.)

SUGGESTED FILLINGS:

- anything in white sauce such as cooked vegetables, tuna or cooked chicken
- strawberry purée
- fruit salad (fresh or canned)

~

PARTY TIME

Little children enjoy parties but can be overwhelmed by the excitement. A good rule of thumb is to invite the number of children for the age of the child; for example a 4-year-old has four guests. Keep time to a reasonable limit too — an hour of excitement is plenty for a young child. Late morning or lunch time is also best for most children, particularly those still having an afternoon sleep.

Make simple finger foods so that you're not worn out before the party begins. Pieces of fruit and vegetables are easy party foods. Avoid hard vegetables such as carrot sticks, plus hard lollies, nuts and sausages, as children can choke.

Planning the Party

- Decide what type of party you want and where it is to be held. Some alternatives to home are a picnic in the park, barbecue, playgroup and the zoo.
- Decide whether you want to serve lunch or snack foods. Will you need to pack up food to take to another venue?
- Allow 2 pieces of savoury food, one piece of dessert-type food plus birthday cake, and a drink for each child.
- Make sure the party food looks attractive. Cut large pieces of food into small, manageable bits. Serve fruit platters and desserts on pretty paper doilies.

- It's traditional to take home some sweets. Be different — make some fresh popcorn, place a small quantity in party bags and tie with a ribbon. Give each child a bag when leaving. You can also put in balloons, a toy, dried fruits or fruit fingers.
- Stick to your guns and provide tasty, healthy foods. Try these menus:

MENU 1
- Rainbow Sandwiches (page 77)
- Little Meatballs (page 63)
- Fruit Platter (page 77) with Apricot Yoghurt Dip (page 68)
- Pink Spiders (page 80)
- Ice Cream Cake (page 78)

Menu 2

- Snake Sandwiches (page 77)
- Bread Cases (page 76) filled with Chicken Easy (page 65)
- Pizza Wheels (page 67)
- Pikelets with Tasty Toppings (page 68)
- Easy Birthday Cake (page 79)
- Green Bubbles (page 80)

Children from 3 years also enjoy:
- Pieces of cold chicken
- Baked Macaroni (page 71)
- Slice of bread spread with Penny's Pâté (page 67)
- Apple and Custard Tartlets (page 75)

Popcorn is high in fibre and low in fat, making it a tasty and nutritious snack for children.

Snake Sandwiches

Allow half a slice of bread per child. Cut crusts off bread. Roll with a rolling pin and spread with smooth peanut butter. Roll up and cut into four.

~

Summer Fruit Platter

watermelon
rockmelon (canteloupe)
strawberries
Apricot Yoghurt Dip (page 68)

Cut fruit into small pieces and arrange on a wooden platter with the dip in the centre. Allow 2–3 pieces of fruit per child.

~

Oven-baked Fingers

Allow one-third of a slice of bread per child. Lightly spread bread with margarine, sprinkle with grated cheese and cut into three fingers. Place on oven tray and bake at 220°C (425°F) for 10 minutes. Cool on a cake rack.

Small pieces of cold roast chicken are also well liked. You can make a party more sophisticated for older children.

~

Winter Fruit Platter

apples
pears
mandarines
Apricot Yoghurt Dip (page 68)

Cut fruit into small pieces and arrange on a wooden platter with the dip in the centre. Allow 2–3 pieces of fruit per child.

~

Rainbow Sandwiches

white bread
wholemeal bread
avocado
grated carrot
cream cheese

Spread one slice wholemeal bread with mashed avocado. Place white bread on top, lightly spread with margarine, sprinkle with grated carrot, place wholemeal bread on top, spread thickly with cream cheese. Top with a slice of white bread. Trim crusts and carefully cut into three ribbons.

~

Birthday Cakes

ICE CREAM CAKE

PREPARATION TIME: 10 MINUTES

Children love ice cream, so this simple cake is sure to be a winner.

> 1 cup (155 g/5 oz) strawberries, sliced
> 500 g (1 lb) vanilla ice cream

Allow ice cream to soften, then beat with electric mixer, stir in strawberries. Line a pudding bowl with plastic wrap and allow it to overhang the edges. Pour ice cream into bowl and freeze (approximately four hours). Turn onto a serving plate and remove plastic wrap. Place fresh fruit around the base and on the top. Push toothpicks into candles and push these into top of cake. (Remove from freezer about 20 minutes before serving to allow it to soften slightly.)

~

SPONGE CAKE

> ½ sponge cake
> 125 g (4 oz) cream cheese
> fruit, to decorate

Beat cream cheese until creamy consistency. If necessary, thin with 1 tablespoon milk. Split cake, spread half the cream cheese in the middle, replace top of cake and spread remainder of cream cheese on top. Decorate with fruit, such as strawberries, other berries or kiwifruit.

You might also try commercial baby foods, such as fruit, custards, or gels as fillings and toppings for a birthday cake.

~

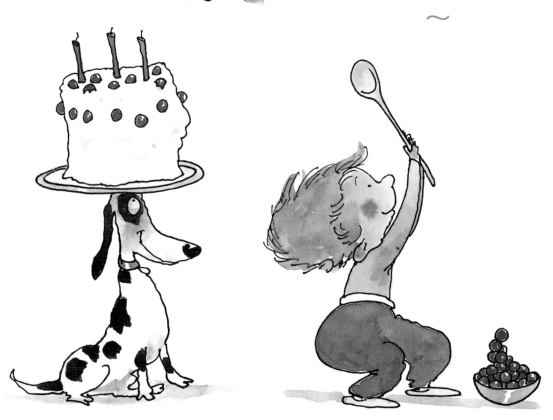

EASY BIRTHDAY CAKE

No party is complete without a lovely birthday cake. This recipe was given to us years ago. It is high in fat and sugar and certainly does not come in the healthy food category, but a small serve for each child is quite acceptable.

1 cup (125 g/4 oz) self-raising flour
1 cup (250 g/8 oz) sugar
½ cup (125 ml/4 fl oz) milk
2 eggs
90 g (3 oz) butter or margarine, melted

Sift flour into mixing bowl and add remaining ingredients. Beat until mixture becomes smooth and thick. Pour into a greased and lined log or round sponge tin. Bake at 180°C (375°F) for 35–40 minutes.

VARIATIONS: Sift 2 tablespoons cocoa with the flour, or add 2 teaspoons grated orange peel.

Cover a piece of stiff cardboard with foil. Place cake in the centre of the board. Cover with Cream Cheese Frosting (see below) and decorate with fresh fruit and, of course, the candles.

 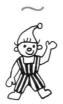

CREAM CHEESE FROSTING

125 g (4 oz) cream cheese
1 cup (155 g/5 oz) icing sugar

Soften cream cheese at room temperature, then process until smooth. Gradually add icing sugar and beat until smooth.

This can be used on cakes or as fillings instead of the traditional icing.

Picnic Parties: In fine weather, make up a small plastic bowl (with lid) with a few sultanas, a slice of cheese, a few strawberries, some popcorn, and two Snake Sandwiches (page 77) for each child. You can sit on a rug under a shady tree and cleaning up couldn't be easier — just shake the rug! In colder weather, try the same idea indoors.

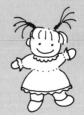

Party Drinks

PINK SPIDERS

MAKES 8–10 SMALL CUPS

1 cup (155 g/5 oz) strawberries, washed and hulled
1 litre (32 fl oz) bottle of soda water
vanilla ice cream

Purée strawberries. Place a tablespoon of purée in each cup, add 2 teaspoons of ice cream and carefully pour soda water over. Stir gently. Spiders will climb up the side of the cup. As the froth subsides a little, top up with a bit more soda.

Don't overfill drinks for small children and make sure everyone is sitting down before serving.

~

GREEN BUBBLES

MAKES 8–10 SMALL CUPS

6 kiwifruit
1 litre (32 fl oz) bottle of soda water

Peel and purée kiwi fruit. Place a tablespoon of purée into each cup and add soda water.

~

APRICOT DREAM

MAKES 8–10 SMALL CUPS

250 g (8 oz) canned unsweetened apricots, drained
¾ cup (200 ml/6 fl oz) plain yoghurt
1 cup (250 ml/8 fl oz) milk

Purée fruit in a blender, add yoghurt and blend, gradually adding milk. Half fill cups and top with a couple of pieces of chopped apricot. Serve each child a cup with a spoon.

This is quite filling and could take the place of dessert.

Most children hate wearing hats — especially party hats! Try brightly coloured ribbons tied around their wrists instead.

~

CHAPTER SIX

A to Z Easy Reference

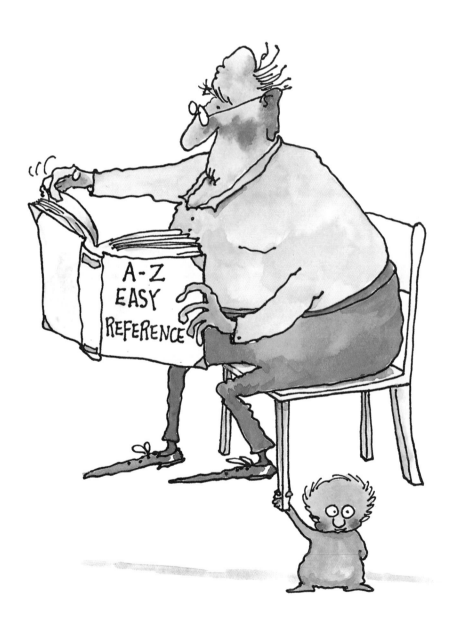

ADDITIVES

Food additives are used to improve food's keeping qualities; it's taste, texture and appearance; to enhance nutritional value; and to assist processing. Additives have been used for centuries, the earliest being salt, sugar, smoke, vinegar and spices. Food additives allow us to have a varied, year-round supply of foods that are safe, wholesome and consistent in flavour, texture, colour and nutritional value. The types, purity and quantities of additives allowed in foods are strictly set out in government Food Standards Codes. Those used must have been shown to be necessary and safe. All food additives are mentioned in the ingredient list, with the class name followed by the name of the additive or its number. A list of approved additive numbers is available from Government departments. The numbering system makes food choices easier for consumers with food sensitivities.

ALLERGY

Food allergy is a reaction some people have to a food protein. The immune system produces antibodies as a defence against the 'foreign' protein, causing symptoms such as swelling, itching, wheezing, vomiting, tummy pains, diarrhoea and eczema. These symptoms usually occur within one to two hours. Foods that can cause such reactions include cow's milk, egg, peanut, fish and soy.

While many parents tend to blame allergies for eating problems in children, it is important to remember that the incidence of true food allergy is very small (less than 10 per cent of children). Food allergy tends to run in families and is most common in small babies and in children where there is a history of known allergy. In addition to family history, reactions also depend on age and the time of exposure to the offending food.

Allergy can occur in young babies introduced to proteins (other than those in breast milk) before 4–6 months. The gut is not fully mature and allows proteins to pass through the gut wall into the bloodstream and reach antibody-forming cells. Continue breast feeding for at least 6 months and delay introducing solids until the recommended times to help avoid allergies.

If there is a history of allergy in the family, continue breast feeding for as long as possible and preferably don't introduce those foods known to cause an allergic reaction until at least 12 months. Breast feeding mothers with a history of allergy may help prevent allergies in their babies by following a diet which excludes the offending foods. Most children tend to grow out of their allergies by 3–4 years of age. If you suspect an allergy, consult your doctor or dietitian for a correct diagnosis and expert dietary advice.

See also *Cow's milk allergy, Eggs, Food intolerance* and *Soy milk*.

ALUMINIUM

A non-essential dietary mineral, we ingest aluminium from foods, drinking water, medications, cooking utensils and aluminium cans. Most is excreted by the kidneys, but it is toxic to the brain, liver and bone if it accumulates and has been implicated in Alzheimers disease. Babies can be at risk of aluminium toxicity due to immature gut and kidney systems. Concern has been raised about the high aluminium content of soy formulas and the use of aluminium-containing antacids for the relief of infant colic.

The aluminium content of soy formulas is considered to be within safe limits.

ANAEMIA

This is the most common nutritional problem among babies and young children worldwide. It is mainly caused by a lack of iron, although it can also be caused by an infection, disease or deficiencies in other nutrients. Anaemia is most likely to happen in children between 6 months and 3 years, when growth rate is rapid and milk is still a major source of kilojoules.

It rarely occurs before 4–6 months because the baby is born with his own iron stores, but once these have been exhausted problems can arise if breast feeding or infant formula is not continued and if iron-containing foods are not included in the diet. This is why you should not continue reduced-iron formula after 4 months. Premature babies are born with lower stores and have a faster growth rate, so they have special iron needs.

Cow's milk is a poor source of iron and should not be used as the main milk source before 9 months and preferably not until 12 months. Iron deficiency during infancy and childhood can have long-term effects. Recent studies show that iron is important for normal nerve and brain development.

To prevent iron deficiency in your baby: breast feed or use an iron-fortified formula until at least 12 months; use infant cereals in preference to adult cereals which are lower in iron; introduce meats (red and white) by 6 months; use vitamin C–containing foods with iron–rich foods to enhance absorption; and do not introduce solids before 4 months. Other good sources of iron for toddlers include baked beans, pork, veal, soy beans, lentils, chickpeas and pâté.

ASCORBIC ACID

Ascorbic acid (vitamin C) is essential for maintaining health especially during growth. It is not stored and needs to be supplied every day. Breast milk (providing the mother's diet is adequate) and infant formula contain adequate amounts of vitamin C. Other sources include citrus fruits (oranges, mandarines, lemons, grapefruit), capsicum (peppers), broccoli, strawberries, mango, tomatoes, potatoes, cabbage and cauliflower.

BACTERIA

These are the microorganisms that occur everywhere, including in the body. Some bacteria are not harmful and have a useful purpose: the bacteria in our gut produce vitamin K (essential for the clotting of blood) and help break down dietary fibre. Other bacteria can be harmful when they multiply to large numbers in food left at room temperature. Some food poisoning bacteria can be fatal. It is important to handle and store food at the correct temperature to keep it safe. Refer to *10 ways to avoid close encounters of the germy kind* on page 30.

BAKED BEANS

These are a popular food for young children and adults. They are made from navy beans which are cooked with various sauces, usually tomato. They are a nutritious, economical food, high in fibre (4.8 per cent), protein (4.6 per cent) and complex carbohydrate: low in fat, (0.5 per cent) and cholesterol-free. They make an excellent meat substitute in vegetarian diets and for children who do not like eating meat. Baked beans can be introduced into your baby's diet from 6 months. Mash or purée to begin with, and choose salt-reduced varieties.

BETA CAROTENE

A naturally occurring yellow/orange pigment in plants, beta carotene is important because it can be converted into vitamin A in the intestine. It is found in dark green leafy vegetables (such as spinach, cabbage and lettuce), carrots, pumpkin, broccoli, orange, mangoes, apricots, red capsicum (pepper) and tomatoes. Unlike vitamin A, beta carotene is not toxic if eaten in large quantities.

BISCUITS

Savoury biscuits can make a healthy snack for kids. Choose low or reduced-salt and wholemeal varieties. Sweet biscuits can be included occasionally to meet the increased energy needs of children and for variety. Too many can have an adverse effect on teeth, and prevent your child from enjoying other foods.

BRAN

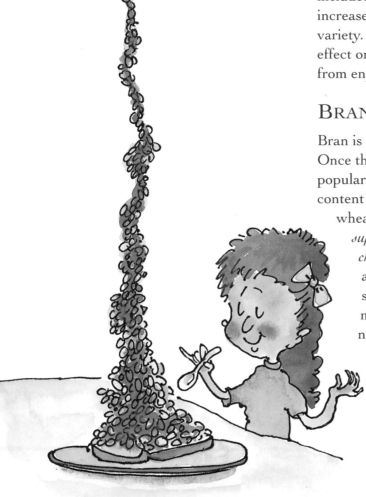

Bran is the outer layers of cereal grains. Once thrown out as waste, it is now popular as a way of increasing the fibre content of diets. Common brans include wheat, oats, barley and rice. *Bran supplements are not recommended for children.* They can decrease the absorption of necessary minerals such as calcium, iron, zinc and magnesium; fill up the child, leaving no room for more important foods needed for growth and development; and they may have a scouring effect on the bowel, causing bleeding. Babies and children should get enough fibre from foods such as wholegrain breads and cereals, fruits and vegetables and legumes.

BREAD

All breads — whether, white, mixed grain, wholemeal or ryes — are nutritious foods. Bread supplies protein, complex carbohydrate, dietary fibre, vitamins (particularly thiamin) and minerals. Bread can be introduced into your baby's diet from 6 months.

CAFFEINE

This is a naturally-occurring stimulant to the nervous system, found in coffee, tea, cola beverages, cocoa and some drugs. It is retained longer in the pregnant woman's body before excretion in the urine. It crosses the placenta during pregnancy and stays even longer in the unborn child, who has no enzyme to break it down.

Babies born to mothers who had a high caffeine intake during pregnancy have been shown to exhibit withdrawal symptoms for 1–2 weeks after the birth.

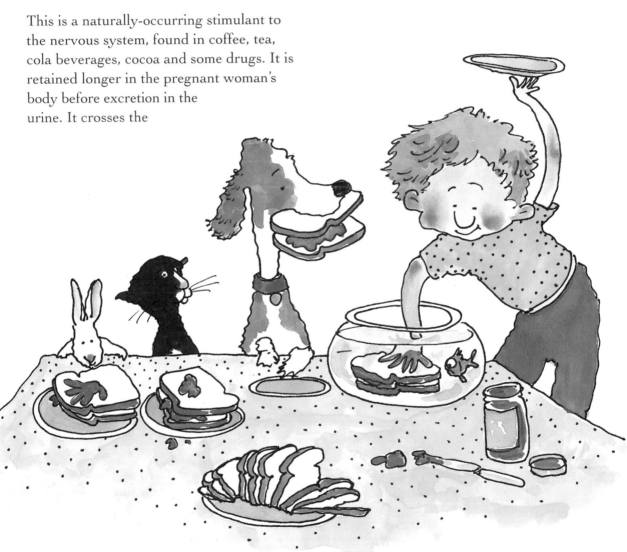

The effect of caffeine on babies and children is largely unknown, but studies have shown no link between a normal intake (4 cups of coffee daily) during pregnancy and birth defects or developmental problems. Caffeine also passes into breast milk but there is no evidence that it has an effect on a baby's sleep.

CALCIUM

Calcium is needed for teeth and bones, blood clotting, blood pressure and for the correct functioning of nerves and muscles. The main sources are dairy foods. Some calcium is also found in fish with bones (sardines, salmon), vegetables (broccoli, parsley, cabbage), legumes, almonds and oranges, but it is not as well absorbed from these foods as it is from milk. Tofu (bean curd) is a good source of calcium, but unfortified soy milk is not. For children, only use soy milks which have calcium added to the same level as that of cow's milk. Skim milk and reduced fat milks contain the same or slightly more calcium than whole cow's milk. Lack of calcium early in life can increase a person's chances of getting osteoporosis later. Calcium is particularly important during pregnancy and breast feeding.

A child's daily calcium needs will be met by 200 ml (6 fl oz) milk plus 200 g (6 oz) of yoghurt and a wedge of cheese (40 g/1½ oz), or by 600 ml (18 fl oz) milk.

CALORIES

See *Energy*.

CARBOHYDRATES

These provide energy for the body. There are two forms — simple and complex. Simple carbohydrates are sugars such as glucose, fructose, galactose, maltose, sucrose and lactose. Complex carbohydrates include starches and dietary fibre. Glucose is the main fuel for the brain; most sugars and starches are ultimately converted into glucose in the body. Most fruits, vegetables, cereals, breads, legumes and nuts contain a mixture of simple and complex carbohydrates. Most simple carbohydrates (sugars) are found in fruit, vegetables, sugar cane, milk, honey and jam, while most complex carbohydrates (starches) are found in bread, cereals, grains, vegetables (such as potato and corn) and legumes. Health authorities recommend we eat a diet high in complex carbohydrates. See also *Energy, Starch,* and *Sugar*.

CHOLESTEROL

Cholesterol is a white fatty substance made in the liver and is an important part of the membranes of the brain and nerves. Breast milk is a high-cholesterol food, which shows just how important cholesterol is for babies. Cholesterol is not found in plant foods. A high blood cholesterol level in adults is a result of the liver over-producing cholesterol together with a diet high in saturated fat (hard fats such as butter, cream, fat on meat, and fats in cakes, biscuits, pies and pastries); it is not caused simply by eating high cholesterol foods. However, children should not be given a low-fat, low-cholesterol diet without the supervision of a dietitian or doctor as nutrients required for growth and development may be omitted.

CHOKING

Choking can occur when food or objects get stuck in the throat, or by the inhalation of foods or liquids into the lungs. It is a life-threatening situation and babies are particularly at risk because everything gets put into their mouths. Common foods causing choking are hotdogs, lollies, nuts, grapes, whole peas, bits of apple and raw carrot. To help prevent choking:
• always watch your child when eating
• do not let your child 'eat on the run'
• do not give hard pieces of fruit, vegetables, cheese or meat until your baby is ready to chew them — blanch, grate or mash them instead
• remove skins, seeds and pips from fruit
• do not give sausages, nuts, whole peas, raw carrots, bubble gum or lollies to a baby
• remove all bones and skin from meats and fish
• watch 'nibbles' put out for guests when your toddler is around
• do not leave small objects such as buttons, crayons, pins, needles, beads or marbles on floors and tables

Ask your baby health nurse for advice on first aid for choking.

COLIC

Colic is a common problem, very distressing for parents and difficult to define. A colicy child has been described as one who is healthy and well fed, but has sudden attacks of irritability, fussiness or crying lasting for more than three hours per day and occurring on more than three days in any one week. A baby with colic cannot be settled, and many reasons have been claimed, including food allergy, wind, infections, tummy upsets and emotional factors in the mother or baby. Some paediatricians say it should be more correctly called 'crying' or 'fussing' and, because it is quite common (about 60 per cent of babies), they say it is a natural developmental stage many babies go through as a result of the changes occurring in their nervous system. This offers little comfort!

Some breast feeding mums find their babies are more settled if they exclude spicy foods, cabbage, broccoli, coffee and onions from their diets. However, changing formula for bottle fed babies does not appear to help. Colic appears to start at about 6 weeks and usually stops by 3 months. Crying seems to be worst in the evening when parents are tired and least able to cope. Parents should remember that professional advice is available from various organisations. Ask your baby health nurse or paediatrician for a referral. Fortunately, this stage does pass!

COLOSTRUM

See page 10.

COMMERCIAL BABY FOODS

See page 31.

CONSTIPATION

This refers to the hardness of the 'poos' rather than frequency.

Causes include:
• lack of dietary fibre (in children over 12 months)
• lack of water
• lack of exercise
• emotional stress (such as starting a new kindergarten)
• too busy playing — children often 'hold back' and ignore the need to use their bowel
• incorrect mixing of formula in bottle fed babies.

To prevent/relieve constipation:
• increase the fibre in the diet (in children over 12 months)
• add maltogen to formula
• add more fluid to the diet
• use prune juice or stewed prunes
• encourage your child to go to the toilet when 'nature calls'
• when all else fails, soft licorice works wonders for young toddlers!

If these efforts fail, see your doctor as medical treatment may be needed. See also page 23 for more information on constipation in bottle fed babies.

COW'S MILK

See page 16.

COW'S MILK ALLERGY

Many parents seem to think their child has an allergy to cow's milk, but in fact less than 10 per cent of the child population has a true allergy. It is most common in babies breast fed for only a few weeks and then given cow's milk-based formula. The porous, immature intestine allows the protein of cow's milk to enter the circulation and produce antibodies. Soy and goat milks

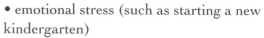

are not suitable substitutes in many cases as there can be a further reaction to these proteins; at least two thirds of babies allergic to cow's milk will also be allergic to goat's milk.

Many people also claim that milk causes mucus congestion and cough. However, studies have not shown an association between dairy products and mucus production — the physical effects are not caused solely or specifically by milk.

DEHYDRATION

Dehydration is loss of water from the body, and means that essential body functions cannot be performed. Dehydration is usually caused by diarrhoea and vomiting and in extreme cases, can lead to death. Young babies and children can quickly become dehydrated. Signs of dehydration include weight loss, thirst, lethargy, sunken eyes, low blood pressure, little or no urine output (very few wet nappies) and skin that retracts slowly when pinched. Always check with your doctor if you suspect dehydration in your child.

See also *Water*.

DIARRHOEA

This is the frequent passing of very loose bowel motions and is often associated with vomiting and tummy pains. It can be caused by bacteria (such as food poisoning), viruses (as in gastroenteritis), infections of urinary or respiratory tracts, food intolerance, antibiotics and some medical conditions such as diabetes. Diarrhoea is the body's way of getting rid of an offending toxin; in the process water

and important body minerals (electrolytes) are lost. Loss of too much water (dehydration) and minerals can cause death, so in the treatment of diarrhoea the aim is to prevent dehydration. The following guidelines are for babies and children who are not dehydrated.

In breast fed babies under 12 months with diarrhoea, continue breast feeding but give extra clear fluids as suggested below, diluted with cool boiled water. For bottle fed babies under 12 months, stop the formula for 24 hours and give electrolyte solutions (as a first preference) or the other clear fluids suggested below. Again, use cool boiled water for diluting. Reintroduce formula at half-strength for the next 24 hours, three-quarter strength for the next 24 hours and then full strength.

In young children over 12 months with diarrhoea, stop food for the first 12–24 hours and give clear fluids only. Suitable fluids include:
• electrolyte solutions available from chemists (e.g. Gastrolyte, Electrolade, Glucolyte — follow manufacturer's instructions);
• cordials (not low joule) diluted 1:6 in tap water;
• unsweetened fruit juice or fruit juice drinks diluted 1:4 with tap water;
• carbonated drinks (not low joule), diluted 1:4 with warm water to eliminate bubbles;
• glucose — 2 teaspoons in 1 cup (250 ml/8 fl oz) cool boiled water.

Your child will need about 5–7 ml per kilogram of weight per hour of fluids. So for a 3 year old weighing 14 kg (7 lb) this is about 70–100 ml/hour or 240 ml (8 fl oz) every 2nd hour.

If you feel diarrhoea may be caused by the drinking water, use cool boiled water for diluting.

Cordials and carbonated drinks must be diluted as the sugar may cause diarrhoea. Food should be introduced within 24 hours even if diarrhoea has not settled. Some foods which are tolerated after 12–24 hours include potato, pasta, rice, noodles, vegetables, plain biscuits, bread, toast, meat, eggs, fish and soup (not milk-based). Milk products, sugary foods (jelly, honey, jam), dried fruits and fruit should be avoided for a few days as initially they may exacerbate the diarrhoea. In some cases, when milk is reintroduced diarrhoea may start again or become worse. This may be due to a temporary inability to handle milk sugar (lactose), so a suitable low-lactose milk should be used.

'Toddler diarrhoea' can also occur in young children when they drink too much fruit juice or eat too much fruit, particularly those varieties with more fructose than glucose such as apples, prunes, and pears. Artificially sweetened drinks and fruit juice concentrates containing added sorbitol may also cause diarrhoea. To prevent this, always dilute juice with water (at least to half-strength) and limit to two drinks per day. Encourage your child to have fruit rather than juice. Whole fruit has the same nutrients but is higher in fibre so more filling.

Insufficient fat in the diet can also be a cause of diarrhoea. Check that your child is having a well-rounded intake of food and not too many fruits and sugary foods.

Always consult your doctor for the appropriate treatment of diarrhoea in your child.

Clean hands, clothes and kitchen will also help prevent diarrhoea. See also *Dehydration.*

EGGS

Eggs are a nutritious food containing protein, fat, vitamins A, B, D and E and the minerals calcium, phosphorus, potassium, zinc and iron (although the iron is poorly absorbed). The only missing major nutrients are fibre and vitamin C. One egg contains about 355 kJ (85 cal). Eggs have been criticised for their high cholesterol content, but saturated fat in the diet contributes more to blood cholesterol than the actual cholesterol content of food. Children can eat an egg a day where there is no history of heart disease or high cholesterol in the family. For adults with a normal blood cholesterol level, one egg per day in conjunction with a reduced-fat diet is also acceptable. See also *Fats.*

Egg yolk is usually introduced into the diet at about 6 months of age. Egg yolk protein is rarely allergenic but, as with all new foods, should be served well-cooked and introduced gradually in case there is a reaction. Egg yolk protein is desensitised by heating, as with commercial egg custard.

Egg white is more allergenic than egg yolk and should not be introduced until about 9 months. It contains little fat and cholesterol. If there is a known history of egg allergy, delay the introduction of egg till after 12 months.

ENERGY

Energy is the ability to do work and is needed by the body for physical activity, body temperature maintenance, metabolism and growth. Because they are growing rapidly, babies need a high energy intake. Energy comes from the breakdown of food and is measured in kilojoules or calories. (One calorie is equivalent to 4.2 kilojoules.) Fats have twice the kilojoules of proteins and carbohydrates, so foods high in fat have a high energy content. In most Western countries we derive too much of our food energy from fats; most should come from carbohydrates.

See also *Carbohydrates* and *Fats*.

FAT BABIES

Being big or plump does not mean your baby is fat or overweight. During the first six months of life, 60 per cent of the weight he gains will be fat, 20 per cent over the first year. Remember these important points:

• You can't tell if your baby is fat just by looking at him. Visit your local baby health nurse regularly to check that he is growing and his weight is in proportion to his height.

• Exclusively breast fed or formula fed babies (under six months) will not be fat/overweight if they are not overfed. (Don't misinterpret a cry as always wanting a feed, make formula up correctly and don't insist baby finishes his feed if he clearly shows you he has had enough. Babies have excellent appetite control.)

• Introducing solids too early (before 4 months) will provide extra kilojoules which baby may not need and which may cause a weight increase.

• Most babies gain some fat near the end of the first year; this is usually lost with growth and activity.

• Heredity plays an important part in whether your baby is fat. If mum and dad

are fat, baby may also be fat (see also *Fat children*).

• Fatness in the first 12 months does not mean your baby will be overweight as a child or adult.

• Never put a baby on a strict diet. This may endanger growth and development. Talk to your baby health nurse if you are concerned.

• Encourage your baby to be active after 6 months or when he is ready to crawl, walk and explore. Don't always sit him in the stroller, bouncinette or chair.

FAT CHILDREN

Children become fat when their food intake is greater than their needs. Fat children often suffer emotional unhappiness and teasing which can affect their personality, as well as cause health problems later in life. Prevention is much better than cure, so ensure your child eats sensibly. Avoid high fat and high sugar snacks and encourage exercise.

Some facts to keep in mind:

• As with babies, you cannot tell if a child is fat just by looking at him. Children — especially toddlers — have round faces and protruding stomachs which do not mean they are overweight. See your dietitian or baby health nurse who will check your child's weight against height.

• Not all fat children eat more than normal weight children. Research has shown that heredity plays a part, and that some fat children may inherit genes that make them good storers of fat. It is estimated that if one parent is obese, the likelihood of the child being overweight as an adult is about 40 per cent; if both parents are obese the likelihood is 80 per cent.

- An early increase in the size and number of fat cells between birth and 2 years may also contribute to overweight. Children who are obese at 2 years have more and bigger fat cells than normal weight children.
- Overweight between 6 and 11 years is a good indicator as to whether a child will be an overweight adolescent.
- Strict diets are out for children as they may affect growth, and can lead to emotional and psychological trauma.
- With children, the aim is to maintain current weight or prevent weight gain, not to reduce weight. As the child grows taller, keeping his weight constant will bring him into the ideal weight range.
- Set a good example for the child with healthy family eating habits. Do not have lollies, chocolates, cakes, crisps and so on in the house. These can be allowed occasionally in very small portions when others are having them on special occasions — the child must feel 'normal'.

See also *Obesity*.

FATS

Fats are an important energy source, containing twice the kilojoules of the other sources, carbohydrates and proteins. Fats are a major source of energy for babies and breast milk contains 50 per cent of its energy as fat. Fats are made up of fatty acids and glycerol. Fatty acids can be saturated, monounsaturated or polyunsaturated. Saturated fatty acids are found mainly in animal foods such as eggs, meat, milk and butter, while polyunsaturated fats (safflower/sunflower/soy/maize oils) and monounsaturated fats (canola/olive/peanut oils, avocado) are mainly in vegetable foods. Breast milk contains the right fatty acid balance for a baby. See also *Low-fat diets* and *Monounsaturated fatty acids*.

FIBRE

There are two types of fibre: soluble fibre is found in fruits, vegetables, legumes, rice, barley and oats and is useful in lowering cholesterol, while insoluble fibre is found in wheat, wheat bran and wheat-based foods and is useful in relieving constipation. Fibre is not found in animal foods. Fibre also slows

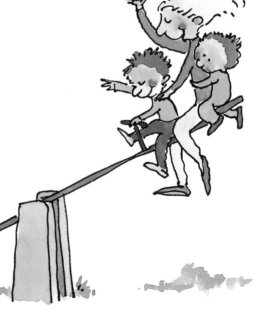

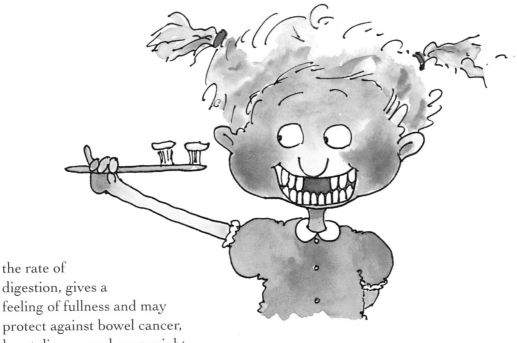

the rate of
digestion, gives a
feeling of fullness and may
protect against bowel cancer,
heart disease, and overweight.
Bran-based adult cereals are not
recommended for babies under one
year. Too much cereal fibre can prevent
adequate intake of energy as it is very
filling and the baby only has a small
stomach capacity. Fibre can also prevent
certain minerals from being absorbed.

FLUORIDE

A natural element important in the
prevention of tooth decay, fluoride
combines with calcium, phosphorus and
other elements to form enamel which is
hard and resistant to decay by bacteria.
Fluoride is particularly important when
teeth are forming and it is absorbed into
enamel. In many areas of the world the
water supply is fluoridated to one part per
million. Since the introduction of
fluoridated water, the incidence of tooth
decay in children has declined
significantly. Formula made up with
fluoridated water will contain adequate

fluoride for a baby. Breast milk is not a
good source of flouride, as fluoride does
not pass into mum's milk.

Supplementary fluoride (0.25 mg/day)
is recommended for breast fed babies
living in unfluoridated areas. It is not
necessary in fluoridated areas, provided
the baby is not exclusively breast fed past
6 months; by this stage he will receive
enough fluoride from the solids and other
fluids in his diet.

If you live in an area with
unfluoridated water, it is suggested that
you prepare at least three litres of
fluoridated drinking water daily and use
this for making up formula, drinking and
cooking. Fluoridated water and foods
prepared with it, plus the use of fluoride
toothpaste, meet adults' fluoride needs. It
should also be noted that some home water
filters remove fluoride.

Folic acid (Folate)

Folic acid is needed for growth and repair of body tissues, and is involved in making blood cells and in fat metabolism. It is found in green leafy vegetables (spinach, broccoli, Brussels Sprouts), yeast extracts, liver, wholegrain cereals, nuts and peanut butter. Fresh goat's milk has little folate and is unsuitable for babies — only goat's milk formula should be used.

A diet rich in folic acid is recommended for pregnant women as a preventative measure against neural tube defects in the baby.

Food intolerance

Many people confuse food allergy with food intolerance: the latter does not involve the immune system nor is it a reaction to protein. It is a reaction to an excessive intake of certain natural or added chemicals. These include salicylates, amines (in cheese, chocolate, fish, yeast extracts, bananas, avocadoes, tomatoes), monosodium glutamate (MSG), food additives such as tartrazine and sulphites. Symptoms of food intolerance are similar to an adverse drug reaction, including tiredness, tummy pains, diarrhoea, hives and headaches. Children usually become irritable, restless and difficult to handle. Food intolerance is difficult to diagnose as it usually involves more than one food and reactions are not always immediate. See your doctor or dietitian if you suspect a food intolerance. See also *Monosodium glutamate (MSG)*, *Salicylates*, *Sulphur dioxide* and *Tartrazine*.

Formula

See page 15.

Fructose

Fructose is also called 'fruit sugar' as it is found in all fruits and honey. It is also a component of sucrose (table sugar), but 1½ times sweeter. Fructose is not completely absorbed by young children and a high intake may cause wind, bloating, cramping and diarrhoea. Always dilute fruit juices and limit intake to 1 to 2 serves daily.

Fruit juice

Fruit juice is a source of vitamin C (plus small amounts of other vitamins and minerals). It is mainly carbohydrate (sugar), with little fat or dietary fibre. Juice is usually used as a fluid source rather than for its vitamin C, which is already adequate in breast milk and formula. 'Fruit juices' are made from 100 per cent fruit juice, while 'fruit juice drinks' have 25–50 per cent juice and 'fruit drinks' 5–25 per cent juice. All commercial juices contain added vitamin C. Fruit juices should be diluted to half-strength for babies and young children.

Fussy eaters

Children usually start to become fussy eaters after 12 months and are fussiest between 18 months and 2 years as they become active, independent toddlers. Fortunately the stage does pass! See Chapter 4.

GASTROENTERITIS

This is a viral or bacterial infection of the stomach and intestine causing diarrhoea, vomiting and tummy pains. It can be life-threatening if it leads to dehydration. See *Dehydration* and *Diarrhoea.*

GLUCOSE

Glucose is the most important sugar in the body, being the major source of energy for the brain and nervous tissue and the form in which carbohydrate is circulated in the blood. Starch and most sugars (with the exception of fructose) are broken down to glucose before absorption.

GLUTEN

Gluten is a complex protein found mainly in wheat, but also in smaller amounts in rye, oats and barley. It is the gluten in wheat flour which gives bread its raised structure and light texture. Gluten is also used as a binder in sausages and smallgoods. Children and adults with coeliac disease must avoid foods containing gluten.

GOAT'S MILK

Goat's milk is unsuitable for babies under 12 months unless in the form of an infant formula. Goat's milk is low in folic acid and vitamins B6, B12, C and D. Raw goat's milk should never be given to babies and young children. Goat's milk is often recommended for cow's milk protein allergy, but at least two-thirds of children who are sensitive to cow's milk will also be sensitive to goat's milk.

HERBAL TEAS

Because herbal teas can contain naturally-occuring toxic substances (the hygiene and purity of the tea may also be questionable), they should be used with caution during pregnancy and breast feeding and for babies and young children. During pregnancy, the chemicals in herbal teas cross the placenta (as do alcohol, tobacco and caffeine). While these chemicals are relatively harmless to mother, they may have an adverse effect on the unborn child. Similarly, the chemicals in herbal teas which pass into breast milk can affect a baby. Remember that small amounts of a herb can have a signigicant effect on a baby's small body. Some mothers use chamomile to settle colic in young babies, but it should never be used for babies with a family history of allergy as it is known to cause an allergic reaction.

HONEY

Honey is the sweet syrup made by bees from the nectar of flowers. It contains about 75 per cent sugars (glucose and fructose) and 25 per cent water. Honey is often used as a sugar substitute on the assumption that it contains more nutrients. While this is true, you would have to eat about 11.2 kg to get your requirements for calcium, 4 kg for iron and 0.5 kg for zinc! Honey, like all sugars, can cause tooth decay. Because it can contain clostridium botulinum spores which cause food poisoning and which are not destroyed by heating or processing, honey is not recommended for babies under one year. Botulism in babies can cause constipation, breathing problems, paralysis and even death.

HYPERACTIVITY

Hyperactive children have a short attention span, poor concentration, are hard to discipline, uncoordinated, throw tantrums, have unpredictable behaviour and generally can't control themselves. Much controversy has surrounded the link between diet and hyperactivity. In 1975, Dr Ben Feingold of the Kaiser Research Institute, San Francisco, claimed a dramatic improvement in 50 per cent of children when salicylates and artificial colours and flavours were eliminated from their diet. The 'Feingold diet' has now been widely challenged, criticised, and largely disproved. However, various food sensitivities have been found in some hyperactive children. Other research linking refined sugar foods with hyperactivity has also been disproved.

More recent studies indicate a link between low iron levels (anaemia) in babies and hyperactivity. Iron is important for the proper growth and development of the brain.

IODINE

Iodine is necessary for growth and is required by the thyroid gland (at the base of the throat) to produce thyroxin which controls the body's metabolism. Iodine is found in iodised salt, seafood, vegetables and dairy products. Lack of iodine can cause goitre (characterised by very large swelling in the neck). It is toxic in large doses. Supplements are generally not necessary.

IRON

See *Anaemia*.

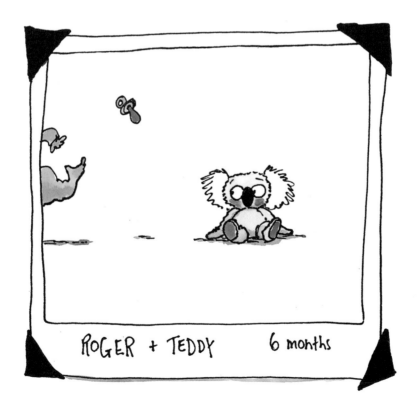

ROGER + TEDDY   6 months

KILOJOULES

See *Energy*.

LACTOSE

This is the sugar of milk and is broken down by the enzyme lactase into glucose and galactose before being absorbed. Babies are born with mature lactase levels to break down the lactose in breast milk (and infant formula). Breast milk and infant formula contain about twice the lactose content of cow's milk, so are very sweet. Lactose is the least sweet of all the sugars.

LACTOSE INTOLERANCE

This is a condition where lactose (milk sugar) is not broken down to glucose and galactose due to a lack of enzyme lactase. Some babies are born without lactase, but this is rare. Lactose intolerance most commonly occurs temporarily after gastroenteritis but can also occur with other diseases such as coeliac disease. Some young babies are unable to completely digest lactose, and this has been suggested as a possible cause of colic. Lactose intolerance is common in certain population groups, including Australian aborigines, American blacks, Indians, Greeks and many Asian groups.

The lactase enzyme disappears after about 3 years of age in these groups, so they can only tolerate small amounts of dairy products after that.

Symptoms of lactose intolerance include watery, explosive diarrhoea, tummy pains and wind. Treatment involves a diet free from milk and dairy foods with a substitution of lactose-free or low-lactose milks. Soy milks or infant soy formulas are usually suitable.

LAXATIVES

Used by adults to relieve constipation, laxatives may contain bulking agents such as gums or chemicals which affect the wall of the bowel. Laxatives are not recommended for babies and children except on the advice of a doctor. They can cause uncomfortable tummy pains, loss of water and a general weak feeling.

See also *Constipation*.

LEAD

Lead is a toxic mineral in the body. Children are particularly vulnerable to lead poisoning because they absorb more lead than adults. Lead can come from food, air pollution (particularly car exhaust fumes), dust and leaded paint. Lead poisoning affects the brain so that learning difficulties can occur.

LECITHIN

Lecithin is a fatty substance found naturally in eggs, legumes, wholegrains, chicken, meats and oils. It is used as an emulsifier in processed foods to prevent the separation of fat. The body also makes its own lecithin which is important in fat metabolism.

LEGUMES

Legumes are a good and economical source of protein, complex carbohydrate, dietary fibre, vitamins and minerals. They are also low in fat. Legumes include all dried peas and soy/butter/haricot/lima/kidney/navy beans and lentils. Baked beans made from navy beans are a favourite with young children and are an excellent meat substitute. All beans (except canned) need to be soaked before cooking and boiled rapidly for 5–10 minutes. The boiling helps kill any toxins present in legumes.

LOW-FAT DIETS

These are not recommended for children under 5 years. Fats are important for a child's growth and development, for fat-soluble vitamins and cholesterol (for hormones and brain and nerve tissue).

A poor fat intake can also lead to diarrhoea (particularly if excessive fruit and juice is taken). Vegan children are particularly at risk. Fat for children should be obtained from whole cow's milk and other dairy products, eggs, lean meats, fish and small quantities of margarine/butter. High-fat foods such as biscuits, crisps, pastry items, doughnuts and fried foods should only be served occasionally. Where there is a family history of heart disease or high blood cholesterol, the child's diet should be managed with the supervision of a dietitian. See also *Fats*.

LOW-FAT MILKS

These are milks which have some of the fat removed. Compared with whole cow's milk at 4 per cent fat, reduced fat milks have 1–2 per cent fat while low-fat milks such as skim milk have a fat content of 0.1 per cent. Reduced and low-fat milks are not suitable for babies

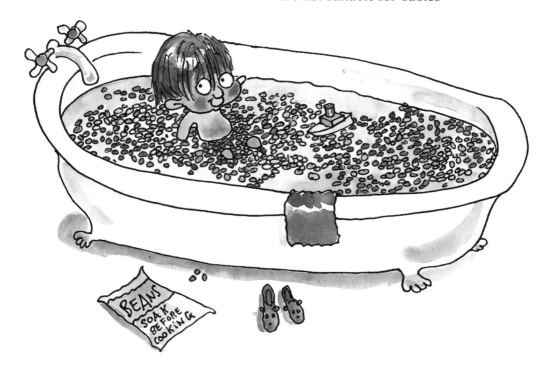

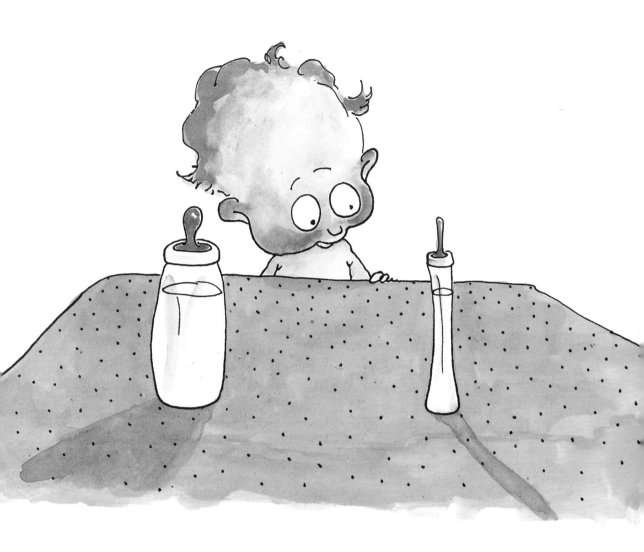

and children under 5 years as the primary milk drink, because they lack the fat, fat-soluble vitamins and energy needed for growth and development.

MICROWAVE COOKERY

Microwaving is a quick and convenient way of heating and cooking foods with little nutrient loss, provided that cooking times are correct. It involves the use of high energy radiation which heats the water particles within the food. Microwaves heat foods from the outside in, and foods keep heating once removed from the oven, so always stir well before serving. See also page 22.

MODIFIED STARCHES

These food starches are made from natural starches such as rice, wheat or maize. They have been modified so that they are stable during food processing. They are used as thickeners and help to maintain consistency and texture. Commercial baby foods use modified maize starch. A baby over 4 months is able to adequately digest starches.

MONOSODIUM GLUTAMATE (MSG)

MSG is the sodium salt of glutamic acid, an amino acid of protein. This acid occurs naturally in meat, fish, breast milk, Parmesan cheese and vegetables such as tomatoes, carrots and corn.

MSG is used as a flavour enhancer in many foods such as soups, sauces and stock cubes. It is not added to baby foods. Some people are sensitive to MSG, but reactions are rarely due to MSG alone, rather they occur in combination with a sensitivity to other food chemicals. MSG sensitivity is characterised by headaches with a tightness or numbness and sensations of burning in the face, neck and chest. It is sometimes described as 'Chinese restaurant syndrome', but an Australian study has found that the glutamate content of Italian meals is much higher than that of Chinese meals! Extensive research worldwide has demonstrated that MSG is safe for human consumption. See also *Food intolerance*.

MONOUNSATURATED FATTY ACIDS

These are found in olives and olive oil, canola oil, avocadoes, lean beef, lean pork, veal, chicken, salmon, tuna, almonds, peanuts, peanut oil and peanut butter. They have recently become popular following research showing they protect against heart disease, lower cholesterol and have a beneficial effect on blood pressure.

NITRATES

Nitrates are present in many foods, the amount depending largely on the soil, as nitrates are a common ingredient in fertilisers. Nitrates are also used as preservatives, colouring and flavouring agents in sausages, salamis, ham, bacon and corned meat.

Nitrates can be a problem to young babies, so cured meats and vegetables such as spinach, beetroot, turnip, kale (collard) and carrot (or juice) should not be given to a baby before 6 months. In babies nitrate is easily converted to nitrite which in turn oxidises the iron of haemoglobin to a compound methemoglobin. Methemoglobin cannot carry oxygen, so that death can occur from respiratory failure. Cases of nitrate poisoning have been documented in babies over-consuming spinach, and cases of mild poisoning from carrots and well water. Vitamin C and vitamin K appear to prevent the conversion of nitrate to nitrite.

NUTRASWEET

Nutrasweet is the brand name for the sugar substitute Aspartame. Aspartame is made from aspartic acid and phenylalanine which individually are not sweet but, when combined, have a sweetening power 180 times that of sugar. Aspartame is metabolised in the body the same way as other protein foods. It is safe for children over 12 months, adults, pregnant and breast feeding women, but is not recommended for those with the genetic disorder phenylketonuria. Aspartame is used in low-joule soft drinks, yoghurts and cordials and in 'light' chocolate.

NUTS

Nuts are a useful source of protein (7–20 per cent), dietary fibre, vitamins B and E and minerals (iron, calcium, zinc, magnesium, potassium and phosphorus). They are very high in fat, ranging from 36 per cent in hazelnuts and coconut to 75 per cent in macadamias. Nuts contain no cholesterol and are low in carbohydrate. Nuts can be processed into flours and pastes. Peanut butter is a nutritious spread for children and adults. Whole nuts should not be given to young children because of the risk of inhalation and choking.

OATS

Oats are a popular cereal grain food which require some processing before being eaten. We buy them as rolled oats, oat bran or oatmeal, but they are also a popular ingredient in foods such as bread, biscuits, breakfast cereals (muesli) and cakes. Oats contain 7 per cent fat, the highest fat content of all the cereal grains. The fat is mainly polyunsaturated and monounsaturated. Oats are a good source of complex carbohydrate and dietary fibre, B vitamins, calcium and iron. Rolled oats are not a suitable infant cereal before 9–12 months because of their high fibre content and lower level of iron compared with specialised infant cereals. The presence of gluten also excludes their use before 6 months.

OBESITY

A child is said to be obese when his weight is 20 per cent more than the average weight for his height on height/weight tables. Obesity is the more extreme form of overweight. See *Fat babies* and *Fat children*.

OESOPHAGEAL REFLUX

See page 24.

OLIVE OIL

A popular oil used in Mediterranean cooking, olive oil is very high in monounsaturated fatty acids which protect against heart disease. It contains no cholesterol. Olive oil has a distinctive strong flavour and greenish colour.

OMEGA 3 FATTY ACIDS

Sources include breast milk, fish (salmon, tuna, mackerel, herring, sardines), egg yolk, lean red meats, pork, canola oil, walnuts and soy beans. They protect against heart disease and stroke, increase bleeding times (so protect against thrombosis), lower blood pressure, may improve arthritis, and may be important in cancer, and asthma prevention. Omega 3 fatty acids are important for babies' nerve and eye development.

PECTIN

A soluble fibre found in citrus peel and other fruits and vegetables, pectin helps jam set and is used as a thickening agent in fruit-flavoured fillings and spreads, confectionery, chutneys, sauces, salad dressings and mayonnaise. It delays the emptying of the stomach and helps to lower cholesterol.

PRESERVATIVES

These are food additives approved under Government regulations to control the growth of moulds, yeasts and bacteria in order to increase the shelf life of foods. In canned, frozen and dried foods, the process is the preservative: commercial baby foods in jars and cans do not contain preservatives.

RECOMMENDED DIETARY INTAKES (RDI)

RDIs are the intakes of vitamins, minerals, protein and kilojoules considered necessary to meet the requirements of healthy people in each age group. RDIs are decided by expert committees. Each country publishes its own RDIs which are available from government bookshops and public health and nutrition departments.

REFLUX, OESOPHAGEAL

See page 24.

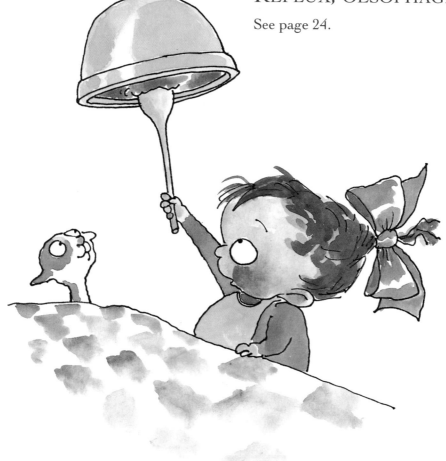

RENNIN

An enzyme produced by the gastric glands, rennin works on casein (a milk protein) by converting it to a curd-like substance which looks like sour milk. Rennin is not produced in adults.

SALICYLATES

These are naturally-occurring chemicals found in many foods including fruits (apples, apricots, blackberries, cherries, peaches, oranges, mandarines), vegetables (carrots, tomatoes, cauliflower, potatoes, pumpkin, turnip, corn, zucchini), nuts, herbs, spices, jams, honey, yeast extracts, tea, coffee, juices, beer and wine. They are also found in perfumes, eucalyptus oils, aspirin and peppermint. Salicylate can cause unpleasant reactions in sensitive people if too much is eaten. See also *Food intolerance*.

SALT

Common table salt is made up of sodium and chloride. People in Western countries consume 8–12 grams of salt per day, when the body requires only half a gram per day. Too much salt in the diet has been associated with high blood pressure, stroke, fluid retention and heart disease. A baby gets enough salt from breast milk and formula and the natural salt content of foods without needing added salt. Babies cannot rid excess salt from their bodies to the same extent as adults — a high intake may cause dehydration as it needs a lot of water for excretion. Most commercial baby foods do not contain added salt. However the salt content of all commercial baby food is low, being strictly controlled by food regulations.

SKIM MILK

This very low-fat milk (0.1 per cent fat) is not recommended for babies or children less than 5 years as it is too low in energy, fat, and the fat-soluble vitamins A and D.

SORBITOL

Used as a sugar substitute in low-joule foods such as jams and chocolates, sorbitol also helps to retain moisture in foods such as baked goods. It occurs naturally in a number of fruits but can also be made synthetically, and is about half as sweet as sucrose. Large amounts of sorbitol (20–50 grams) can cause bloating, wind and diarrhoea. Sorbitol is not completely absorbed by the body.

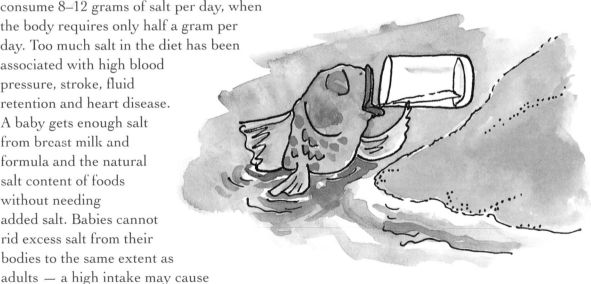

SOY MILK

Made from soy beans which have been soaked, ground, cooked and strained, soy milks contain no lactose and are often used for lactose intolerance and after gastroenteritis. However, in some of these cases a reaction to the soy protein may occur, so it must not be used where there is an allergy to cow's milk protein. For babies less than 12 months old, a soy formula must be used in preference to soy milk, as soy milk is nutritionally inadequate for a baby's growth and development. For children over 12 months where soy milk replaces cow's milk, use a fortified milk similar in composition to that of cow's milk. Compared with cow's milk, unfortified soy milk (or soy drink) is low in calcium, vitamins A, B2 and B12, the amino acid methionine, energy, protein and fat. The presence of certain compounds in soy milks may reduce the absorption of calcium, zinc and iron.

STARCH

Starch is the stored form of glucose in plants. Modified starches from maize or tapioca are used in some infant formula and commercial baby foods; they thicken food on heating and improve the stability of the product. Starches are easily digested to glucose for energy. See also *Carbohydrates*.

SUGARS

Sugars vary in sweetness, the sweetest being fructose, then sucrose, glucose, maltose, and lactose. (Sucrose or 'table sugar' is a carbohydrate made up of glucose and fructose which is naturally present in fruits and vegetables, honey, golden syrup and maple syrup.) Babies have a natural liking for sweet foods — breast milk is about 1½ times sweeter than cow's milk! Too much sugar in the diet can cause tooth decay, overweight and obesity. See also *Carbohydrates*.

SULPHUR DIOXIDE

This is used as a preservative and anti-oxidant, added to fruit drinks, dried fruit, soft drinks, beer, wine and sausages. Reactions to sulphur dioxide can occur in sensitive people. Symptoms include nausea, diarrhoea, and asthma. See also *Food intolerance*.

TARTRAZINE

This is a synthetic yellow colouring added to custard powder, snack foods, confectionery, sauces and preserves. There has been some controversy concerning its association with asthma and hyperactivity in children; however, the number of people with tartrazine sensitivity is small and in general the additive is considered safe to use. The additive number is 102. See also *Food intolerance*.

TEA

Tea contains caffeine and tannins: quantities vary with the strength of the tea. It is not recommended for babies and young children. See also *Caffeine* and *Herbal teas*.

THICKENERS

Thickeners are used to give a thicker consistency to foods to improve 'mouth feel' and prevent separation of foods during processing and storage. Thickeners include vegetable gums and gelatine but are predominantly starches from a variety of sources including corn, wheat, potato and rice. Thickeners are used in some baby foods, sauces, soups, jellies, ice cream and desserts.

UNDERWEIGHT

Children are said to be underweight when their weight is less than what is suitable for their height. Most children said by parents to be underweight are not — they just happen to be thin and small (or tall), often a characteristic seen in the rest of the family. As long as they eat well and are growing and developing normally, there is no need to worry. Check with your baby health nurse or dietitian. On the other hand, a child who is consistently thin and not growing needs attention. Causes might include an underlying illness, emotional problem or poor diet. Growth failure and underweight are seen in children whose parents unnecessarily restrict their diet to prevent overweight by offering very low fat foods and high fibre foods and by cutting out healthy snacks. (See *Low-fat diets*). Vegetarian, particularly vegan, children can be at risk. (See page 40.) Underweight, or failure to thrive, is serious in babies. Regular visits to your baby health nurse or doctor will pick up the problem if it occurs.

VEGETARIAN DIETS

See page 40.

VITAMIN C

See *Ascorbic acid*.

VITAMIN K

This is a fat-soluble vitamin found mainly in green vegetables, liver and soy beans; it is also made by bacteria in the gut. It is important for blood clotting. Newborn babies are given vitamin K by injection or, more recently, as an oral dose, which reduces risk of haemorrhaging and bleeding.

WATER

Water is essential for life. At birth a baby's body contains 75 per cent water; by 4 months water content reaches that of an adult, 60 per cent. Water is needed to maintain fluid balance, for chemical reactions, to transport substances in and out of cells and for the body's secretions and excretions. A baby requires an average of 150 ml/kilogram/day, while children need 1–1½ litres (32–48 fl oz) and adults 1½–2 litres (48–64 fl oz) per day. Water comes not only from what we drink but also from the foods we eat (bread has 40 per cent water, breast and cow's milk 87 per cent, fruit 80–90 per cent and beef 63 per cent), and from the breakdown of carbohydrates, fats and proteins in the body. In very hot humid climates, babies lose water very easily and extra may be needed in the form of extra breast feeds or cooled boiled water. All water for babies under 12 months should be boiled for at least 5 minutes. See also *Dehydration*.

WEANING

This term is used to describe the changing to foods other than breast milk. Some babies wean themselves. Discuss weaning with your baby health nurse.

YEAST

Yeast is a single cell organism related to fungi such as moulds and mushrooms. Yeasts are a good source of protein with little fat and sugar, and a rich source of B vitamins (except B12). They are also high in minerals (potassium, phosphorus, iron, chromium, zinc, selenium, magnesium and calcium). Reactions to yeast and yeast-containing foods occur in some sensitive children. As yeasts also contain salicylates and amines — common natural chemicals causing food intolerance — a diet avoiding yeasts and moulds may not solve the problem.

YEAST EXTRACT

This is a black, salty spread made from yeast and an excellent source of B vitamins. Yeast extracts are also used to boost flavours, but should be used sparingly because of their high salt content.

YOGHURT

Yoghurt is made from pasteurised cow's milk or skim milk mixed with cultures and held at 45°C until it thickens. It is then cooled, flavoured and sweetened. The cultures break down the milk sugar (lactose) to lactic acid, giving yoghurt its characteristic acid taste. This conversion makes yoghurt suitable for some people with lactose intolerance. Yoghurt has the same nutritional properties as milk and

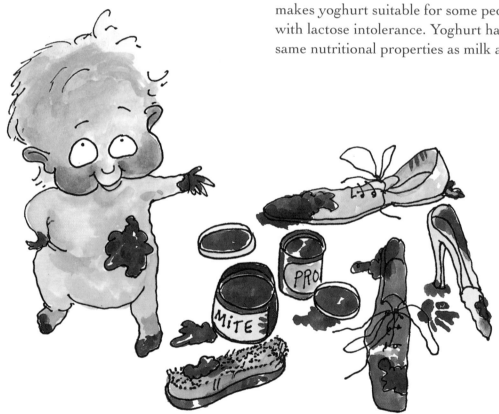

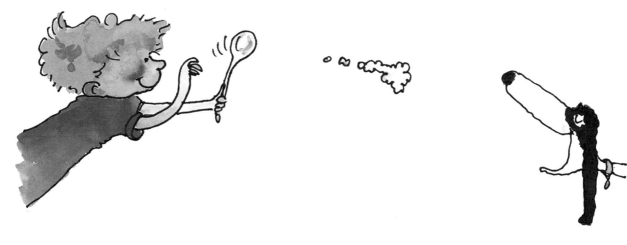

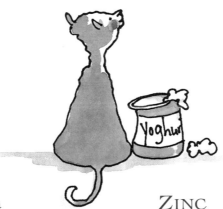

can be introduced to a
baby's diet from
6 months. Yoghurts using the cultures
lactobacillus acidophilus and
bifidobacterium bifidus are becoming
popular as they are said to have many
therapeutic benefits such as improving and
maintaining the natural gut flora,
protecting against gut infection, relieving
constipation and restoring the gut flora
after diarrhoea. Baby yoghurt desserts
contain about 20 per cent yoghurt. The
dessert is sterilised so the yoghurt culture
is destroyed.

ZINC

Zinc is an important mineral found in
lean meat, chicken, cheese, nuts, oysters
and liver. It is important for the body to
enable it to use proteins and carbohydrates
and is essential for wound healing and
good vision. Lack of zinc in the diet can
cause a loss of appetite and taste. Lack
of zinc in children affects growth and
sexual maturity.

INDEX

INDEX *111*

RECIPE INDEX